D1031636

W.B. SAUNDERS COMPANY
A Division of Elsevier Inc.

1600 John F. Kennedy Blvd., Suite 1800, Philadelphia, PA 19103-2899

http://www.theclinics.com

NEUROLOGIC CLINICS
May 2006
Editor: Donald Mumford

Volume 24, Number 2
ISSN 0733-8619
ISBN 1-4160-3576-1

Copyright © 2006 by Elsevier Inc. All rights reserved. No part of this publication may be reproduced or transmitted in any form or by any means, electronic or mechanical, including photocopy, recording, or any information retrieval system, without written permission from the Publisher.

Single photocopies of single articles may be made for personal use as allowed by national copyright laws. Permission of the publisher and payment of a fee is required for all other photocopying, including multiple or systematic copying, copying for advertising or promotional purposes, resale, and all forms of document delivery. Special rates are available for educational institutions that wish to make photocopies for non-profit educational classroom use. Permissions may be sought directly from Elsevier's Rights Department in Philadelphia, PA, USA: phone: (+1) 215 239 3804, fax: (+1) 215 239 3805, e-mail: healthpermissions@elsevier.com. Requests may also be completed on-line via the Elsevier homepage (http://www.elsevier.com/locate/permissions). In the USA, users may clear permissions and make payments through the Copyright Clearance Center, Inc., 222 Rosewood Drive, Danvers, MA 01923, USA; phone: (978) 750-8400, fax: (978) 750-4744, and in the UK through the Copyright Licensing Agency Rapid Clearance Service (CLARCS), 90 Tottenham Court Road, London WIP 0LP, UK; phone: (+44) 171 436 5931; fax: (+44) 171 436 3986. Other countries may have a local reprographic rights agency for payments.

Reprints. For copies of 100 or more of articles in this publication, please contact the Commercial Reprints Department, Elsevier Inc., 360 Park Avenue South, New York, New York 10010-1710. Tel.: (212) 633-3813, Fax: (212) 462-1935, e-mail: reprints@elsevier.com.

The ideas and opinions expressed in *Neurologic Clinics* do not necessarily reflect those of the Publisher. The Publisher does not assume any responsibility for any injury and/or damage to persons or property arising out of or related to any use of the material contained in this periodical. The reader is advised to check the appropriate medical literature and the product information currently provided by the manufacturer of each drug to be administered to verify the dosage, the method and duration of administration, or contraindications. It is the responsibility of the treating physician or other health care professional, relying on independent experience and knowledge of the patient, to determine drug dosages and the best treatment for the patient. Mention of any product in this issue should not be construed as endorsement by the contributors, editors, or the Publisher of the product or manufacturers' claims.

Neurologic Clinics (ISSN 0733-8619) is published quarterly by Elsevier. Corporate and editorial offices: 1600 John F. Kennedy Blvd., Suite 1800, Philadelphia, PA 19103-2899. Accounting and circulation offices: 6277 Sea Harbor Drive, Orlando, FL 32887-4800. Periodicals postage paid at Orlando, FL 32862, and additional mailing offices. Subscription prices are $180.00 per year for US individuals, $290.00 per year for US institutions, $90.00 per year for US students, $225.00 per year for Canadian individuals, $340.00 per year for Canadian institutions, $235.00 per year for international individuals, $340.00 per year for international institutions and $120.00 for Canadian and foreign students/residents. To receive student/resident rate, orders must be accompanied by name of affiliated institution, date of term, and the *signature* of program/residency coordinator on institution letterhead. Orders will be billed at individual rate until proof of status is received. Foreign air speed delivery is included in all *Clinics* subscription prices. All prices are subject to change without notice. POSTMASTER: Send address changes to *Neurologic Clinics*, W.B. Saunders Company, Periodicals Fulfillment, Orlando, FL 32887-4800. **Customer Service: 1-800-654-2452 (US). From outside of the US, call 1-407-345-4000.**

Neurologic Clinics is also published in Spanish by Nueva Editorial Interamericana S.A., Mexico City, Mexico.

Neurologic Clinics is covered in *Current Contents/Clinical Medicine, Index Medicus, EMBASE*/Excerpta Medica, and *PsycINFO*, and *ISI/BIOMED*.

Printed in the United States of America.

GUEST EDITOR

RANDOLPH W. EVANS, MD, Clinical Professor of Neurology, Department of Neurology and Neuroscience, Weill Medical College of Cornell University, New York, New York; Department of Neurology, The Methodist Hospital, Houston, Texas; Clinical Associate Professor of Neurology, Baylor College of Medicine, Houston, Texas

CONTRIBUTORS

KAREN E. ANDERSON, MD, Assistant Professor, Departments of Neurology and Psychiatry, University of Maryland School of Medicine, Baltimore, Maryland

J. D. BARTLESON, MD, Associate Professor of Neurology, Mayo Clinic College of Medicine, Rochester, Minnesota

JAY R. BHATT, MD, Assistant Professor of Neurology, Indiana University School of Medicine, Indianapolis, Indiana

PAUL W. BRAZIS, MD, Professor of Neurology and Ophthalmology, Mayo School of Medicine, Mayo Clinic, Jacksonville, Florida

LOUIS R. CAPLAN, MD, Professor in Neurology, Beth Israel Deaconess Medical Center, Department of Neurology, Division of Cerebrovascular Disease; Harvard Medical School, Boston, Massachusetts

MICHAEL CHEN, MD, Stroke Fellow, Beth Israel Deaconess Medical Center, Department of Neurology, Division of Cerebrovascular Disease; Harvard Medical School, Boston, Massachusetts

MICHEL A. CRAMER BORNEMANN, MD, Assistant Professor, Department of Neurology, University of Minnesota Medical School, Minneapolis, Minnesota; Minnesota Regional Sleep Disorders Center, Hennepin County Medical Center, Minneapolis, Minnesota

RANDOLPH W. EVANS, MD, Clinical Professor of Neurology, Department of Neurology and Neuroscience, Weill Medical College of Cornell University, New York, New York; Department of Neurology, The Methodist Hospital, Houston, Texas; Clinical Associate Professor of Neurology, Baylor College of Medicine, Houston, Texas

EDWARD FAUGHT, MD, Professor and Vice Chairman, Department of Neurology, University of Alabama School of Medicine; Director, University of Alabama at Birmingham Epilepsy Center, Birmingham, Alabama

ELLIOT M. FROHMAN, MD, PhD, Professor and Director, Multiple Sclerosis Program, Department of Neurology, University of Texas Southwestern Medical Center, Dallas, Texas

ANDREW G. LEE, MD, Professor of Ophthalmology, Neurology, and Neurosurgery, The University of Iowa Hospitals and Clinics, Iowa City, Iowa

MARK W. MAHOWALD, MD, Professor, Department of Neurology, University of Minnesota Medical School, Minneapolis, Minnesota; Minnesota Regional Sleep Disorders Center, Hennepin County Medical Center, Minneapolis, Minnesota

BOBY VARKEY MARAMATTOM, MD, DM, Department of Neurology, Lourdes Hospital, Kochi, Kerala, India

MICHAEL J. OLEK, DO, Associate Professor, Multiple Sclerosis Program, Department of Neurology, University of Texas Southwestern Medical Center, Dallas, Texas

ROBERT M. PASCUZZI, MD, Professor of Neurology, Indiana University School of Medicine, Indianapolis, Indiana

BRIAN C. SALTER, MD, Resident, Department of Neurology, University of Maryland School of Medicine, Baltimore, Maryland

RONALD SCHONDORF, PhD, MD, Associate Professor, Department of Neurology, Sir Mortimer B. Davis Jewish General Hospital, McGill University, Montreal, Quebec, Canada

MICHAEL SHARPE, MD, FRCP, FRCPsych, Professor of Psychological Medicine and Symptoms Research, School of Molecular and Clinical Medicine, University of Edinburgh, Western General Hospital, Edinburgh, Scotland

WIN-KUANG SHEN, MD, FACC, Professor of Medicine, Mayo Medical School, Mayo Clinic, Rochester, Minnesota

JON STONE, MB, CHB, MRCP, Consultant Neurologist and Honorary Senior Lecturer, Department of Clinical Neurosciences, School of Molecular and Clinical Medicine, University of Edinburgh, Western General Hospital, Edinburgh, Scotland

WILLIAM J. WEINER, MD, Professor and Chairman, Department of Neurology, University of Maryland School of Medicine; Director, University of Maryland Parkinson's and Movement Disorders Center, Baltimore, Maryland

EELCO F. M. WIJDICKS, MD, Division of Critical Care Neurology, Department of Neurology, Mayo Clinic College of Medicine, Rochester, Minnesota

DOUGLAS A. WOO, MD, Clinical Fellow, Multiple Sclerosis Program, Department of Neurology, University of Texas Southwestern Medical Center, Dallas, Texas

CONTENTS

low back pain in a year and among working age people, approximately 50% admit to back symptoms. Neck and upper limb symptoms are less common but may be worrisome because of concern about spinal cord involvement. Many health care providers are uncomfortable dealing with spine and limb pain because of multiple possible causes; concern about loss of neurologic function; cost of evaluation and treatment; and workers' compensation, legal, and medicolegal concerns. This article's cases describe common spine syndromes, when to consider investigation and consultation, and appropriate treatment options.

FORTHCOMING ISSUES

RECENT ISSUES

THE CLINICS ARE NOW AVAILABLE ONLINE!

Access your subscription at
www.theclinics.com

ELSEVIER
SAUNDERS

NEUROLOGIC
CLINICS

Neurol Clin 24 (2006) xi–xii

Preface

Neurology Case Studies

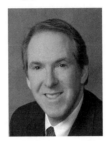

Randolph W. Evans, MD
Guest Editor

Why bother with case-based reviews? We could just publish another *Clinics* of articles centered around evidence-based medicine. However, in clinical neurology, we treat patients one at a time and then try to apply evidence-based medicine. At times, the history, physical, or diagnostic testing may not fit into neat little diagnostic categories. Often, results from Class I studies are inconclusive, or the patient does not fit the study criteria. There is so much nuance in how we diagnose and treat. The art of medicine is alive and well in neurology practice. If evidence-based medicine were computer software, we'd currently be using version 2.0.

In addition, actively working through case studies is, for us, akin to the use of flight simulators for pilots. I suspect we learn much more from case studies than we do from review articles, because we first consider each case as though he/she were our own patient, then we come to our own conclusions and compare them to those of the subspecialty experts who review the latest evidence and give their opinions.

This issue of the *Neurologic Clinics* reviews cases and topics in cerebrovascular disease, multiple sclerosis, syncope, neuromuscular disorders, sleep disorders, epilepsy, spine disorders, neuro-ophthalmology, headache, movement disorders, functional symptoms, and critical care neurology. The disorders range from the rare to the mundane, and the issues range from the most controversial to those widely accepted. The authors enjoyed preparing their manuscripts. We hope this issue will educate and, perhaps, even entertain you.

0733-8619/06/$ - see front matter © 2006 Elsevier Inc. All rights reserved.
doi:10.1016/j.ncl.2006.02.001   *neurologic.theclinics.com*

I thank our distinguished contributors for their outstanding articles. I also thank Donald Mumford, the *Neurologic Clinics* developmental editor, and the Elsevier production team for an excellent job. Finally, I am grateful for the support of my wife, Marilyn, and our children, Elliott, Rochelle, and Jonathan.

Randolph W. Evans, MD
1200 Binz #1370
Houston, TX 77004, USA

E-mail address: rwevans@pol.net

ELSEVIER
SAUNDERS

NEUROLOGIC
CLINICS

Neurol Clin 24 (2006) 181–198

Neurology Case Studies: Cerebrovascular Disease

Michael Chen, MD*, Louis R. Caplan, MD

*Beth Israel Deaconess Medical Center, Department of Neurology,
Division of Cerebrovascular Disease, 330 Brookline Avenue, Palmer 132,
Boston, MA 02215, USA*

Case 1: Spontaneous Recanalization of a Symptomatic Occluded Internal Carotid Artery

Case Presentation

An 80-year-old right-handed man was found by his wife as she returned home from work to be sitting in a chair. He did not answer any of her questions and appeared to have a facial droop on the right. The wife relates that about a week prior to this, he told her of transient right-hand weakness with difficulty lifting a cup of coffee.

On examination, he was mute, yet able to follow simple commands. He appeared frustrated while trying to answer questions. He had a right facial droop with a right arm drift. Imaging revealed an acute infarct in the territory of the left superior middle cerebral artery branch (Fig. 1). Imaging of the intracranial vasculature showed no flow signal in the left carotid artery on time-of-flight MR angiography, suggesting occlusion (Fig. 2). There was reconstitution of portions of the middle cerebral artery from collaterals from the left posterior communicating artery as well as branches from the left external carotid artery. The left anterior cerebral artery filled by way of the anterior communicating artery. An ultrasound of his extracranial vasculature showed the patient's left carotid artery to be occluded, whereas his right carotid artery showed 60% stenosis. His transthoracic echocardiogram was normal.

The patient's past history included coronary artery disease and a coronary artery bypass graft in 1989. His lipids were elevated, and he had slight hypertension, which was well controlled with a single agent over the past 5 years.

---

* Corresponding author.
  E-mail address: chenm888@yahoo.com (M. Chen).

0733-8619/06/$ - see front matter © 2006 Elsevier Inc. All rights reserved.
doi:10.1016/j.ncl.2006.01.009

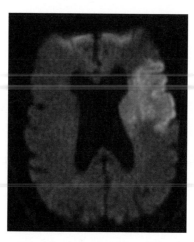

Fig. 1. Diffusion-weighted MRI with restricted diffusion in the territory of a branch off the superior division of the left middle cerebral artery.

At 3 months follow-up, he had a repeat carotid ultrasound performed to assess for changes in his right carotid artery disease. Although the right side was unchanged, there was trickle flow within the left internal carotid artery with peak systolic velocities of 331 cm/s compared with 81 and 186 cm/s for the common carotid artery and external carotid arteries respectively. A CT angiogram at the time showed spontaneous recanalization of the left internal carotid artery with improved flow intracranially (Figs. 3 and 4). There was heterogeneous plaque at the proximal left internal carotid artery at its origin extending approximately 10 mm distally.

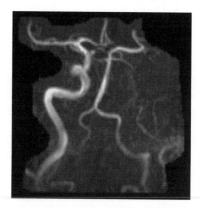

Fig. 2. Magnetic resonance angiography shows no signal within the left carotid artery, suggesting occlusion. There is reconstitution of portions of the middle cerebral artery from collaterals from the left posterior communicating artery as well as probable branches of the left external carotid artery. The left anterior cerebral artery fills via the anterior communicating artery.

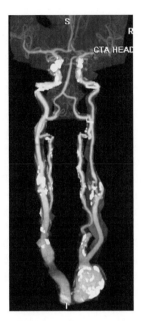

Fig. 3. CT angiography showing partial recanalization of the left internal carotid artery distal to a severe stenosis at the left common carotid bifurcation. There is extensive atheromatous plaque involving the area of stenosis as well as more proximally along the posterior wall of the common carotid bifurcation.

Clinical Questions

Three months after his first infarct, the patient showed spontaneous recanalization of a previously occluded artery ipsilateral to his stroke. Despite the severity of his expressive aphasia, it is a isolated deficit. His comprehension, other cognitive functions, strength, and sensation were spared. The overriding question is whether his left internal carotid artery should be

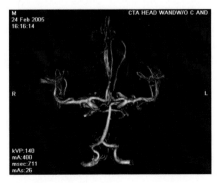

Fig. 4. CT angiography shows patent intracranial vasculature with good flow in the internal carotid artery on the left.

revascularized. His previous occlusion complicates the decision and raises concern for his future risk for stroke and for the risks associated with revascularization.

Discussion

There are few studies about the pathogenesis of an occluded internal carotid artery. Thrombotic occlusion of the coronary arteries has been more clearly described and is generally believed to follow rupture or endothelial erosion of an unstable atherosclerotic plaque [1]. This unstable coronary plaque is characterized by a large core of extracellular lipid or necrotic cellular tissue covered by a thin fibrous layer [2]. The relevance of the coronary plaque instability paradigm to understanding carotid plaques is unclear, but may have some relevance.

In 1969, Fieschi and Bozzao reported the "disappearance" of a distal ICA occlusion on follow-up cerebral angiogram obtained after 3 weeks [3]. One clinicopathologic study looked at 14 autopsies of patients with fatal ICA occlusion and showed thrombus overlying an ulcerated, unstable, atherosclerotic plaque in six of seven occluded carotid sinuses. Several had ipsilateral siphon occlusion. They estimated the underlying plaque without thrombus to cause anywhere from 50% to 95% stenosis, suggesting a possibility for spontaneous recanalization [4]. An acute intraplaque hemorrhage could underlie a temporary occlusion at the site of the plaque, which would then show recanalization over the course of just a few days.

The frequency of spontaneous recanalization of a previously occluded ICA has mostly been anecdotally reported. Reports range anywhere from 17% to 67% and appear to increase with increased time between initial occlusion and follow-up arteriogram [5]. The time course from occlusion to spontaneous recanalization has not been well defined. There are reports of spontaneous recanalization within 1 to 2 hours of onset [3].

CT angiography (CTA) is a rapid, safe, and minimally invasive method that is highly sensitive and specific in diagnosing severe carotid stenosis and occlusion [6]. Particularly in following patients with apparent carotid bifurcation occlusion on duplex ultrasound, CTA is sensitive for distinguishing hairline residual ICA lumen ("string sign") from a true total vascular occlusion. One could argue that CT angiography during the initial presentation may have revealed severe stenosis, and that what was first observed on MRA and carotid ultrasound may have been pseudo-occlusion. But even if the symptomatic carotid artery did have severe stenosis instead of occlusion, the size of the infarct would have required postponement of carotid revascularization for several weeks.

There is controversy over the proper management of near occlusion of the carotid artery. Some advocate emergency endarterectomy, while others caution that revascularization is dangerous. Because patients in the prospective North American Symptomatic Carotid Endarterectomy Trial

(NASCET) trial with high-grade stenosis showed an increasing risk of stroke with increasing deciles of stenosis, patients with near occlusion may have been at the highest risk. A subgroup of patients (7.6% of 3,024 patients) in NASCET with near occlusion of the ICA was studied. ICAs with near occlusion were defined as having greater than 95% stenosis, but nearly all had evidence of robust collateral circulation to the relevant territory. Only a third of patients in the 70% to 94% stenosis group had intracranial collaterals. In NASCET, the presence of near occlusion did not impose an additional perioperative risk, which was at 6.3% [7]. Of the medically treated patients, the 1-year risk of stroke was 35.1% for patients with 90% to 94% stenosis, but was only 11.1% for the patients with near occlusion. The absolute risk reduction at 2 years was 7.9%. This is a more muted benefit than for patients with 90% to 94% stenosis and similar to the degree of benefit found in those patients with 70% to 89% stenosis. One hypothesis behind the drop in stroke risk for patients with near occlusion is that the nearly occluded arterial luminal diameter is associated with markedly reduced pressure such that any embolus formed would have little chance of being carried distally [7].

It is unclear how best to extrapolate the information gleaned from the NASCET subset of nearly occluded ICAs to that of previously occluded ICAs with spontaneous recanalization. What supports the decision to pursue carotid revascularization was that the patient's annual risk of stroke could be interpreted as 11.1%, and there was still a significant portion of his left hemisphere functioning well and at risk for future strokes. The presence of sufficient collateral intracranial flow also decreases the risk for complications such as a hyperperfusion syndrome. Despite his age, the authors felt that his future risk for stroke was significant such that the benefits of revascularization would likely outweigh the risks of the procedure (Fig. 5).

Case 2: An Apparent Intracerebral Hemorrhage and an Unusual Cause of Stroke

Case Presentation

A 78-year-old right-handed woman was noted by her daughter to be speaking strangely over the telephone. Her daughter noted that she seemed confused, inattentive, and mumbling a lot, though able to state a few words clearly and appropriately. Upon arrival at a local community hospital, her speech improved. She stated that she was temporarily confused but felt better. A CT scan of the head (Fig. 6) was obtained, which showed a 1.5 × 1.5 cm circular hyperdense lesion within the right frontal parasagittal cortex adjacent to the falx cerebri with surrounding edema but little mass effect. Anticonvulsant therapy was initiated, and the patient was transferred to the hospital with a diagnosis of a spontaneous intracerebral hemorrhage.

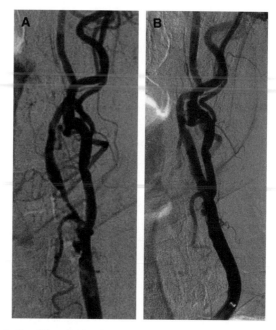

Fig. 5. Carotid angioplasty and stenting pre- (*A*) and poststenting (*B*).

On examination, the patient had diminished attention but normal orientation, language, calculation, and recall. She could draw a full clock and regarded both sides equally well. The remainder of her cranial nerves, motor, sensory, reflex, and coordination testing was normal.

The CT scan was repeated, and the results were unchanged. Further note was made of vasogenic edema surrounding the hyperdensity, suggesting

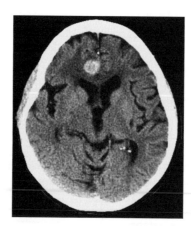

Fig. 6. A noncontrast head CT shows a 1.5 × 1.5 cm circular hyperdense lesion within the right frontal cortex adjacent to the falx cerebri with surrounding edema but little mass effect.

a hemorrhage into a mass lesion. A calcified lesion, such as a meningioma, was also considered.

The leading diagnosis was a single hemorrhagic cerebral metastatic lesion with an unknown primary. A chest, abdomen, and pelvic CT scan were done, and the results were normal.

An MRI with contrast was performed and revealed two small areas of infarction in the territory of the left anterior cerebral artery (Fig. 7A, B). This, combined with the findings on gradient-echo sequence and those with gadolinium, suggested the possibility of a partially thrombosed aneurysm arising from the anterior cerebral artery (Fig. 7C, D). The location of the infarcts suggested the left as opposed to the right anterior cerebral artery to harbor the aneurysm.

A conventional angiogram (Fig. 8A, B) confirmed the presence and location of a partially thrombosed 4 × 6 mm aneurysm at the branch point of the left pericallosal and callosomarginal branches of the left anterior cerebral artery. The wide neck made endovascular coiling problematic and

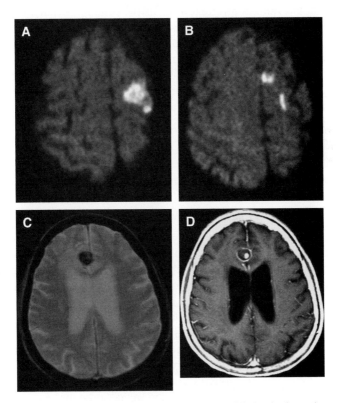

Fig. 7. MRI of the brain shows two small areas of restricted diffusion in the territory of the left anterior cerebral artery along the high convexity of the left frontal lobe (*A, B*) and a susceptibility blooming artifact was seen on gradient-echo sequences (*C*). There is a thin peripheral enhancement after administration of gadolinium as well as central enhancement (*D*).

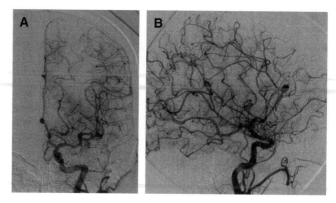

Fig. 8. Conventional cerebral angiogram showed a wide-necked 6 × 4 mm aneurysm at the branch point of the pericallosal and callosomarginal arteries of the left anterior cerebral artery. AP (*A*) and lateral (*B*) views are shown.

justified further evaluation to determine if the benefit of such a complicated procedure truly outweighed the obvious risks.

Although there was no subarachnoid blood on CT scan of the head, a lumbar puncture was performed to determine if there was any blood in the cerebrospinal fluid (CSF), which would indicate that this aneurysm had ruptured. Because the CSF showed no blood or xanthrochromia, her unruptured aneurysm was managed medically and followed with serial exams.

Clinical Questions

What is the mechanism for stroke in this patient? How does the presence of the cerebral embolic events from an untreated aneurysm affect management?

Discussion

The rounded, well-demarcated hyperdensity seen on CT scan was mistaken for a spontaneous intracerebral hemorrhage. The location was atypical for a hemorrhage resulting from chronic hypertension or amyloid angiopathy. The distinctive features included the rounded shape, surrounding vasogenic edema, and lack of significant mass effect. On CT, aneurysms typically appear as rounded lesions of increased radiodensity compared with normal brain and markedly enhance with IV contrast medium [8]. These unusual features to the hyperdensity on CT scan should have raised the suspicion for an aneurysm earlier, and may have prevented the delay in diagnosis and the ordering of unnecessary testing, such as the chest, abdomen, and pelvic CT scan.

Only a handful of case reports have described in any detail the phenomenon of cerebral emboli originating from intracranial aneurysms. A retrospective review over a 10-year period at the Mayo clinic further shows the low incidence of this process. Ninety-seven patients with less than 1-cm aneurysms treated surgically were examined and only 15 (15.5%) presented with symptoms other than rupture. Of these 15 patients, only five had symptoms of cerebral ischemia originating from the aneurysm [9].

It is often difficult to establish an aneurysm as the cause of a stroke or mere coincidence. Cohen et al [10] suggest four criteria by which to determine if cerebral ischemia is the result of embolization from an aneurysm: (1) clinical TIAs or complete stroke; (2) arteriographic, surgical, or autopsy verification of the aneurysm; (3) no other lesions present that could cause produce TIAs or stroke; and (4) no clinical or radiographic evidence of recent subarachnoid hemorrhage or vasospasm or alternative etiology [10].

Several mechanisms have been proposed to explain cerebral ischemia from unruptured intracranial aneurysms. Taptas and Katsiotis in 1968 [11] first proposed the possibility of emboli from the aneurysmal sac. They described a patient who developed right hemiplegia and aphasia 15 days after subarachnoid hemorrhage. Angiography at the time showed a round filling defect in the left carotid artery just distal to the origin of the posterior communicating artery. This filling defect was postulated to result from the thrombus in the aneurysm [11]. Hoffman and colleagues found fresh thrombus in the aneurysmal sac at operation [12]. Antunes and Correll obtained more detailed pathologic information from an autopsy case showing an aneurysm harboring a mural thrombus with a partially organized clot protruding into the parent artery lumen [13].

Another mechanism proposed involves compression or displacement of the parent artery or adjacent arteries by the aneurysm. This was the mechanism initially believed to explain how the paramedian mass could cause strokes in the territory of the contralateral anterior cerebral artery. Mehdorn et al described a patient with TIAs secondary to direct compression of the parent vessel [14].

A history of TIAs in the corresponding territory of an aneurysm, or evidence as in the authors' patient of cerebral infarcts from an aneurysm, suggests the presence of intraaneurysmal clot. To prevent fresh emboli during either endovascular coiling or surgical clipping, some authors recommend temporary proximal and distal parent vessel occlusion. If the definitive treatment is surgical, the clot can be removed once the sac is opened, and subsequent clipping can then be performed with less risk [15]. If endovascular coiling is to be performed, particularly in cases of large or wide-neck aneurysms, where the thromboembolic rate is already higher from the procedure itself, aggressive antithrombotic agents should be considered before or during treatment [16].

Because of the aneurysm size, presence of partial thrombosis, and unruptured state, the primary clinical concern was not rupture but more embolic complications. Because of the wide aneurysm neck and distal location of the aneurysm, coiling would be technically challenging and may not necessarily be more effective than medical management. The authors opted to reimage the patient after a week to assess for acute expansion and observe her while on anticoagulation. If she had no evidence of expansion acutely, the risk of rupture was likely acceptably low. If there were no further embolic events during monitoring for a week, then medical management was likely sufficient.

Case 3: Acute Stroke in a Young Woman

Case Presentation

A 32-year-old woman was finishing a certification exam when she noted, promptly at noon, the acute onset of dizziness and headache. The headache was described as right-sided, throbbing, and retro-orbital. As she looked up from her test paper when the time was up, she noticed that she could not see things on the right side. She covered each eye independently and noted the same problem in both eyes. There was no preceding bright light, and she did not have a history of migraine headaches.

On examination, her blood pressure was 118/70 and her pulse was 80 and regular. On neurologic examination she had a complete right hemianopia. There was some ataxia and loss of fine finger movements on her right side. A head CT was normal. There was restricted diffusion in the territory of the left posterior cerebral artery (PCA) involving the lateral thalamus. MR angiography was remarkable for a cutoff at the left inferior P2 branch. MRA of the neck was normal but did not include T1-weighted images with fat saturation.

She arrived at our hospital at 4 hours after onset of symptoms, and it was decided that despite the NIHSS of only 2, the hemianopia was sufficiently disabling such that the risks associated with intraarterial thrombolysis was outweighed by the possible benefit of restoring her vision on the right side, especially with such a clear vascular lesion on MR angiography to pursue.

Selective catheterization of the left vertebral artery showed a filling defect of a P2 branch of the left PCA (Fig. 9A, B). A total of 20 mg of tPA was used in addition to 2,000 U of heparin. Postprocedure angiogram showed recanalization of the previously occluded P2 branch of the left PCA (Fig. 9C, D). Near the end of the procedure, she reported a worsened headache. An immediate CT scan of the head was performed after the procedure and was remarkable for a hyperdensity for hemorrhagic transformation of the left occipital lobe infarct (Fig. 10A). Protamine was administered and her family was informed of the hemorrhagic complication.

Fortunately, upon arrival to the intensive care unit, her headache was easily treated and vision in the left inferior quadrant improved. A head CT scan the following morning showed interval disappearance of the hyperdensity in the region of the left PCA, indicating that this hyperdensity was

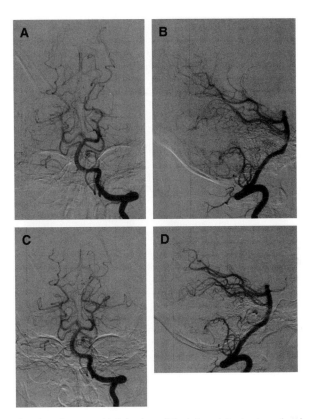

Fig. 9. Conventional angiogram with injection of the left vertebral artery showing a filling defect at the left proximal P2 segment on A/P (*A*) and lateral (*B*) views. After intraarterial thrombolysis with 20 mg of tPA, partial recanalization is seen in the left P2 segment on A/P (*C*) and lateral (*D*) views.

contrast and not blood. No new regions of hemorrhage were seen (Fig. 10B).

She was found to have a patent foramen ovale on transesophageal echocardiogram with right-to-left shunt during rest and with maneuvers. A cardiothoracic surgery was consulted to evaluate for PFO closure. During the next few days of her hospitalization, she had some clumsiness with her right leg. She felt compelled to stare at the ground when she walked and felt dizzy if she were to look straight ahead while walking. She was eventually transferred to an acute rehabilitation facility.

Clinical Questions

This case highlights important clinical issues related to PCA territory infarct localization, acute catheter-based stroke therapy, and stroke management of a young patient with a patent foramen ovale (PFO).

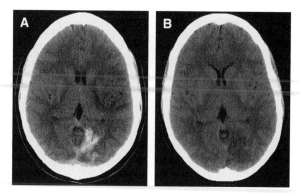

Fig. 10. Noncontrast CT scan performed immediately after intraarterial thrombolysis shows a hyperdensity in the vascular territory supplied by the left posterior cerebral artery suggestive of hemorrhagic transformation (*A*). Noncontrast CT performed the following morning shows only a hypodensity in the left medial occipital lobe, suggesting the previous hyperdensity to be the result of contrast dye during angiography.

Discussion

Occlusion of the posterior cerebral artery is well known to cause homonymous hemi- or quadrantanopias, depending on the extent of occipital lobe infarction. Somatosensory findings associated with PCA territory infarcts have been described by Georgiadis et al in his review of 60 patients [17]. Specific syndromes were described based on the nature of thalamic involvement. Sixteen cases involving patients with lateral thalamic involvement, including infarcts in the territory of the lateral posterior choroidal artery and thalamogeniculate arteries, were discussed. If the thalamogeniculate artery was involved, accompanying minor motor abnormalities, including limb and gait ataxia, were often present. Georgiadis et al concluded that the coexistence of hemisensory symptoms and hemianophia localized the lesion proximal to the lateral thalamus and almost always suggested embolism as the mechanism [17].

The recognition of thalamic involvement may have guided the extent of intraarterial thrombolysis. The entire 20 mg of tPA was administered to the inferior P2 branch supplying the inferior occipital lobe. Perhaps a fraction of the administered tPA should have been injected more proximally to involve the lateral posterior choroidal and thalamogeniculate arteries, which may have helped with the patient's right-sided sensory ataxia.

The hyperdensity on the CT scan after the procedure was misinterpreted as hemorrhagic transformation. The mechanism underlying hemorrhagic transformation probably involves reperfusion of ischemically damaged endothelium, which is less able to maintain the blood brain barrier, permitting the intravascular contents to extravasate into the brain parenchyma. The radiographic appearance consists of high-density foci within previously ischemic areas and is virtually always associated with mass effect [8]. Upon closer inspection of the head CT obtained immediately after angiography, the lack of mass effect suggests benign contrast extravasation rather than hemorrhagic transformation of the infarct.

The patient's future risk of stroke in the context of the PFO presented further clinical challenges. The optimal management of patients with PFO and cryptogenic stroke remains unclear because of difficulty in establishing a cause-and-effect relationship and the lack of randomized clinical trials comparing different therapeutic options. A recent review by Wu et al suggested a management algorithm in deciding which patients should undergo either surgical or percutaneous closure [18]. They identified the following factors that would suggest a need to pursue PFO closure: age of 50 years or less, cryptogenic stroke, large PFO, coexisting atrial septal aneurysm, recurrent neurologic events, valsalva maneuver associated with previous events, failure of anticoagulation therapy to prevent events, intolerance to anticoagulation, and high risk of recurrent deep venous thrombosis, or pulmonary embolus [18].

Case 4: Spontaneous Intracerebral Hemorrhage from Venous Occlusion

Case Presentation

A 51-year-old woman was involved in a low-speed rear-end automobile collision while waiting at a red light 5 days before admission. She was awake and did not hurt her head. She reported neck pain the day after the accident, then a new onset headache 3 days before admission. She does not regularly suffer from headaches. On the day of admission, she vomited once in the morning and was then found in the bathroom face down after her husband heard a loud, unexpected thud. When he found her, she kept repeating, "I need to go to the bathroom." She seemed to respond to his questions appropriately. He called for an ambulance and while en route to the hospital, she was noted by the medics to have a seizure. Upon evaluation at an outside hospital, she was intubated and sedated. After a head CT was obtained, she was transferred to the authors' hospital for further evaluation (Figs. 11 and 12A, B).

Upon examination after extubation and cessation of sedatives, she was awake and had difficulty naming objects and describing specific details in pictures. She had difficulty reading but could write short sentences. She neglected the right side. There was no papilledema. There was slight clumsiness of the right hand and leg. Her neurologic deficits were consistent with a lesion in the left temporal parietal region. The initial thoughts about this hemorrhagic lesion were that it represented a delayed traumatic intracerebral hematoma, otherwise known as "Spat-Apoplexie." A CT angiogram was performed as a screen for the unlikely event that a cerebral aneurysm may have led to this hemorrhagic lesion. The vascular study showed no arterial abnormality but did show a large filling defect in the left internal jugular vein and left transverse sinus (Fig. 13).

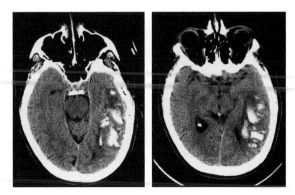

Fig. 11. Noncontrast head CT shows a large, heterogeneous intraparenchymal hemorrhage occupying much of the left temporal lobe, causing mass effect with mild shift of midline structures to the right.

Without evidence that there may be an underlying infection causing the cerebral venous thrombosis, noninfectious causes were investigated. The patient used oral contraceptives and had five miscarriages. Coagulation evaluation showed a slightly low antithrombin III level. Because of her history of seizures, the location and presence of hemorrhage, symptomatic anticonvulsants were started. There was no evidence to suggest increased intracranial pressure by clinical exam and fundoscopy. Despite the amount of acute hemorrhage seen both on CT and MRI, she was treated with heparin followed by coumadin for several months.

Clinical Questions

Does the finding on an occluded left internal jugular and transverse sinus occlusion explain the hemorrhagic left temporal lesion? What predisposed

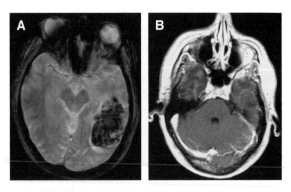

Fig. 12. (*A*) Gradient-echo MRI shows susceptibility artifact occupying much of the left temporal lobe. (*B*) T1 MRI postcontrast shows abnormal signal intensity in the left transverse sinus.

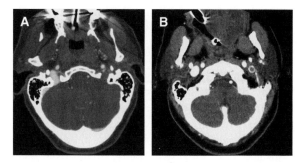

Fig. 13. CT angiography shows an absence of signal in the left internal jugular vein as it exits the skull at the jugular foramen (*A*) and a flow void at the level of the neck (*B*).

this patient to developing the venous occlusion? What is the appropriate treatment?

Discussion

In 1891, Otto Bollinger described four patients who had head injury, followed days to weeks later by death from an apoplectic event. His criteria for the diagnosis of "traumatische Spat-Apoplexie" included the absence of preexisting vascular disease, a definite history of trauma, an asymptomatic interval of at least several days, and an apoplectic episode. Bollinger suggested that cranial trauma caused softening of the brain involving the wall of an artery with eventual rupture of the vessel, necrosis, and hemorrhage after several days [19].

Until the authors obtained imaging of her blood vessels, the patient's clinical picture was consistent with the diagnosis of Spat-Apoplexie with the exception of a definite history of head trauma. She lacked preexisting vascular disease, had an asymptomatic period lasting days, and then an apoplectic episode with apparent hemorrhage into infarcted tissue. Furthermore, there were no identified coagulation abnormalities. It was her CT venogram that showed a clear absence of flow within the left internal jugular vein up to the lateral sinus that established the diagnosis of cerebral venous thrombosis.

The patient presented with an unusual headache, seizures, and then apoplexy. In previously published series of cerebral venous thombosis, headache is the most common symptom, and often is the initial symptom. Other reported symptoms include focal deficits, seizures, altered consciousness, transient visual obscurations, and hemianopia [20]. Because multiple veins are often involved, the inherent variability within the cortical venous system and the rapid development of collateral circulation, clinical syndromes are less well-defined as those described in arterial occlusion.

On imaging, venous infarcts on CT scan manifest as a spontaneous hyperdensity in 10% to 50% of cases. They are often large subcortical, multifocal hematomas or petechial hemorrhages within large hypodensities. This patient's scan was more consistent with the latter characterization. Venous infarcts, as opposed to arterial infarcts, have prominent vasogenic edema and absent or moderate cytotoxic edema [21]. Depending on where the venous occlusion lies, the venous infarct can be seen superficially and paramedian, within the basal ganglia or, as in this patient, over the lateral convexity [21]. Thrombosis of the lateral sinus usually manifests as raised intracranial pressure, with variable involvement of adjacent sinuses. Thrombosis of the internal jugular vein is most often caused by cannulas used for long-term venous access, or more commonly, spread from the sigmoid sinus [22]. Infection involving the skull base may lead to a jugular foramen syndrome, with risks of clot propagation to the superior vena cava and subclavian veins [23].

The etiology of the patient's CVT remained elusive. The incidence of septic CVT has been greatly reduced in developed countries since the introduction of antibiotics and currently accounts for less than 10% of cases [23]. In young women, CVT occurs more frequently during puerperium than during pregnancy. In developed countries, the role of oral contraceptives is more important. Use of oral contraceptives is the only etiologic factor in about 10% of cases, but should be considered more of a risk factor [24]. Among the numerous noninfective medical causes of CVT, congenital thrombophilia is the most common, especially prothrombin gene and factor V Leiden mutation, and prothrombin mutation [25].

The primary issue regarding treatment in such a patient with idiopathic cerebral venous thrombosis is the use of antithrombotics. Jugular vein ligation and surgical thrombectomy have been used in the past but have been largely abandoned. The best evidence of the efficacy of heparin was obtained by a randomized study in Germany. High-dose intravenous heparin was compared with placebo with angiographically documented CVT. After only the first 20 patients, the trial was stopped because of a statistically significant difference in favor of heparin [26]. Metaanalysis of trials looking at anticoagulation in CVT show an absolute risk reduction in mortality of 14% and in death or dependency of 15% [27]. There is ample evidence to suggest that heparin is safe even when CT or MRI demonstrates a hemorrhagic lesion [28]. Patients with dural sinus occlusion are also at risk for pulmonary embolism [29]. When one considers the safety of heparin and the unpredictability of the outcome of patients with CVT, these results reinforce the use of heparin as first-line treatment for CVT. Anticoagulation should then be continued with coumadin for a minimum of 3 months or longer, depending on the presence of a coagulation disorder [30].

Osmotic agents have a role in reducing brain edema in those patients with pseudotumor-like symptoms. Anticonvulsants are also used in patients who develop seizures. Patients with multiple dural sinus occlusions, especially involving transverse sinuses and jugular veins, usually do not do well. Anticoagulants can only prevent extension of thrombosis and are unlikely to open sinuses. In this select group of patients with extensive thrombosis, mechanical and thrombolytic opening of at least one transverse sinus and jugular vein is indicated.

Summary

Data from randomized therapeutic trials often provide little relevant evidence for therapeutic decisions physicians make daily. By illustrating the nuances of these four complex cases involving cerebrovascular disease, the authors stress the importance of more time spent by specialists at the bedside, exploring patients' symptoms and learning their thoughts, fears, biases, and wishes.

References

[1] Davies MJ, Richardson PD, Woolf N, et al. Risk of thrombosis in human atherosclerotic plaques: role of extracellular lipid, macrophage and smooth muscle content. Br Heart J 1993;69:377–81.

[2] Fuster V, Badimon L, Badimon JJ, et al. The pathogenesis of acute coronary artery disease and acute coronary syndromes. N Engl J Med 1992;326:242–50.

[3] Fieschi L, Bozzao L. Transient embolic occlusions of the middle cerebral and internal carotid arteries in cerebral apoplexy. J Neurol Neurosurg Psychiatry 1969;32:236–40.

[4] Lammie GA, Sandercock PAG, Dennis MS. Recently occluded intracranial and extracranial carotid arteries. Relevance of the unstable atherosclerotic plaque. Stroke 1999;30:1319–25.

[5] Yamaguchi T, Minematsu K, Choki J-I, Ikeda M. Clinical and neuroradiological analysis of thrombotic and embolic cerebral infarction. Jpn Circ J 1984;48:50–8.

[6] Anderson GB, Ashforth R, Steinke DE, Ferdinandy R, Rindlay JM. CT angiography for the detection and characterization of carotid artery bifurcation disease. Stroke 2000;31:2168–74.

[7] Morgenstern LB, Fox AJ, Sharpe BL, Eliasziw M, Barnett HJM, Grotta JC, for the North American Symptomatic Carotid Endarterectomy Trial (NASCET) Group. The risks and benefits of carotid endarterectomy in patients with near occlusion in the carotid artery. Neurology 1997;48:911–5.

[8] Osbourn A. Diagnostic neuroradiology. St. Louis: Mosby; 1994. p. 180–1.

[9] Friedman JA, Piepgras DG, Pichelmann MA, Hansen KK, Brown RD, Wiebers DO. Small cerebral aneurysms presenting with symptoms other than rupture. Neurology 2001;57: 1212–6.

[10] Cohen MM, Hemalatha CP, D'Addario RT, Goldman HW. Embolization from a fusiform middle cerebral artery aneurysm. Stroke 1980;11:158–61.

[11] Taptas JN, Katsiotis PA. Arterial embolism as a cause of hemiplegia after subarachnoid hemorrhage from aneurysm. Prog Brain Res 1968;30:357–60.

[12] Hoffman WF, Wilson CB, Townsend JJ. Recurrent transient ischemic attacks secondary to an embolizing saccular middle cerebral artery aneurysm. Case report. J Neurosurg 1979;51: 103–6.

[13] Antunes JL, Correll JW. Cerebral emboli from intracranial aneurysms. Surg Neurol 1976;6: 7–10.

[14] Mehdorn HM, Chater NL, Townsent JJ, Darroch JD, Perkins RK, Lagger R. Giant aneurysm and cerebral ischemia. Surg Neurol 1980;13:49–57.

[15] Sakaki T, Kinugawa K, Tanigake T, Miyamoto S, Kyoi K, Utsumi S. Embolism from intracranial aneurysm. J Neurosurg 1980;53:300–4.

[16] Soeda A, Sakai N, Sakai H, Iihara K, Yamada N, Imakita S, et al. Thromboembolic events associated with Guglielmi detachable coil embolization of asymptomatic cerebral aneurysms: evaluation of 66 consecutive cases with use of diffusion-weighted MR imaging. AJNR Am J Neuroradiol 2003;24:127–32.

[17] Georgiadis AL, Yamamoto Y, Kwan ES, Pessin MS, Caplan LR. Anatomy of sensory findings in patients with posterior cerebral artery territory infarction. Arch Neurol 1999;56:835–8.

[18] Wu LA, Malouf JF, Dearani JA, Hagler DJ, Reeder GS, Petty GW, et al. Patent foramen ovale in cryptogenic stroke. Arch Intern Med 2004;164:950–6.

[19] Elsner H, Rigamonti D, Corradino G, Schlegel R Jr, Joslyn J. Delayed traumatic intracerebral hematomas: "Spat-Apoplexie." Report of two cases. J Neurosurg 1990;72:813–5.

[20] Mohr JP, Choi DW, Grotta JC, Weir B, Wolf PA. Stroke pathophysiology, diagnosis, and management. Philadelphia: Churchill Livingstone; 2004. p. 301–12.

[21] Chu K, Kang DW, Yvon BW, et al. Diffusion-weighted magnetic resonance in cerebral venous thrombosis. Arch Neurol 2001;58:1569–71.

[22] Bousser MG, Russell RR. Cerebral venous thrombosis. London: WB Saunders; 1997.

[23] Ameri A, Bousser MG. Cerebral venous thrombosis. Neurol Clin 1992;10:876.

[24] Bansal BC, Gupta RR, Prakash C. Stroke during pregnancy and puerperium in young females below the age of 40 years as a result of cerebral venous/sinus thrombosis. Jpn Heart J 1980;21:171.

[25] Martinelli I, Sacchi E, Landi G, Taioli E, Duca F, Mannucci PM. High risk of cerebral vein thrombosis in carriers of prothrombin-gene mutation and in users of oral contraceptives. N Engl J Med 1998;338:1793.

[26] Einhaupl KM, Villringer A, Meister W, et al. Heparin treatment in sinus venous thrombosis. Lancet 1991;338:597.

[27] De Bruijn SF, Stam J. for the Cerebral Venous Sinus Thrombosis Study Group. Randomized placebo controlled trial of anticoagulant treatment with low molecular weight heparin for cerebral sinus thrombosis. Stroke 1999;30:484.

[28] Brucker AB, Vollert-Rogenhofer H, Wagner, et al. Heparin treatment in acute cerebral sinus venous thrombosis: a retrospective clinical and MR analysis of 42 cases. Cerebrovasc Dis 1998;8:331.

[29] Masuhr F, Mehraein S. Cerebral venous and sinus thrombosis. Patients with a fatal outcome during intravenous dose-adjusted heparin treatment. Neurocritical Care 2004;3:355–62.

[30] Masuhr F, Mehraein S, Einhaupl K. Cerebral venous and sinus thrombosis. J Neurol 2004;251:11–23.

ELSEVIER
SAUNDERS

NEUROLOGIC
CLINICS

Neurol Clin 24 (2006) 199–214

Diagnosis and Management of Multiple Sclerosis: Case Studies

Douglas A. Woo, MD, Michael J. Olek, DO,
Elliot M. Frohman, MD, PhD*

*Multiple Sclerosis Program, Department of Neurology,
University of Texas Southwestern Medical Center, 5323 Harry Hines Boulevard,
Dallas, TX 75390-9036, USA*

Multiple sclerosis (MS) is the most common disabling neurologic disease in people ages 18 to 60, second overall only to trauma. This prevalence is more than matched by the complexity of the disease, which is compounded by the dearth of definitive evidence to guide clinical decision making and leaves physicians to rely on their judgment and anecdotal experience. This article attempts to illustrate some of the central questions that arise when confronted with patients who have MS and the thought process that uses available evidence and clinical judgment to resolve these dilemmas. Some of the pertinent questions include:

1. Does this patient actually have MS?
2. Should the patient be treated with disease-modifying therapy?
3. How should the patient who exhibits ongoing disease activity (eg, relapses, progression, or MRI lesions) while on disease-modifying therapy be managed?

Patient vignettes are used to illustrate how specific clinical questions may arise, and the subsequent discussions demonstrate how physicians may arrive at a reasonable course of action to manage individual patients effectively.

Patient 1—the clinically isolated syndrome

A 26-year-old, previously healthy woman presents in an office with a 1-week history of horizontal double vision, particularly when she looks to

Dr. Woo's fellowship is supported by a grant from Serono-Pfizer, through the National Multiple Sclerosis Society. Dr. Frohman receives lecture honoraria from Biogen, Teva, and Serono. Dr. Olek receives lecture honoraria from Biogen, Teva, and Serono.
* Corresponding author.
E-mail address: elliot.frohman@utsouthwestern.edu (E.M. Frohman).

0733-8619/06/$ - see front matter © 2006 Elsevier Inc. All rights reserved.
doi:10.1016/j.ncl.2006.01.002

the right. She denies pain, loss of visual acuity, and other neurologic symptoms. Examination reveals an internuclear ophthalmoplegia, the most common syndrome affecting eye movements in MS. The patient's neurologic examination otherwise is unremarkable. Subsequent MRI of the brain and cervical spinal cord are normal with the exception of a lesion in the pontine tegmentum in the region of the medial longitudinal fasciculus. A spinal tap is significant for the presence of oligoclonal bands and elevated immunoglobulin G (IgG) index (1.5; normal, <0.7).

Does this patient have clinically definite multiple sclerosis?

The most current guidelines for diagnosing clinically definite multiple sclerosis (CDMS) arose from the deliberations of the International Panel on the Diagnosis of Multiple Sclerosis and are known as the McDonald criteria [1]. They use a combination of clinical and objective laboratory findings to establish dissemination of disease in time and space, which is the hallmark of MS. In this specific patient, these criteria could be fulfilled by either a second clinical attack or paraclinical evidence of another lesion localizing to a neuroanatomic region that is separate from the medial longitudinal fasciculus, which is demonstrated most reliably with MRI. Oligoclonal bands and elevations in IgG index are nonspecific markers of central nervous system (CNS) inflammation that are described in a multitude of infectious, inflammatory, and neoplastic CNS diseases in addition to MS. In contrast to MRI, these cerebrospinal fluid (CSF) abnormalities cannot be used to establish dissemination in either time or space. Given the absence of a second distinct clinical syndrome and the absence of any other white matter lesions on this patient's imaging studies, the clinician is unable to diagnose CDMS despite the suggestive clinical syndrome and the abnormal CSF findings. Although an analysis of the CSF in this patient would not have altered the ultimate ability to confirm or refute the diagnosis of MS, there is usefulness in assessing CSF to exclude other diagnostic considerations.

What is this patient's risk of developing clinically definite multiple sclerosis?

Although exact conversion rates to CDMS for this specific clinically isolated syndrome (CIS) are not known, observations from long-term follow-up of patients in the Optic Neuritis Treatment Trial suggest that the risk of conversion from optic neuritis to CDMS during 10 years ranges from 22% to 56% [2]. The most important predictor of conversion to CDMS is the MRI finding at symptom onset, where disseminated lesions (in addition to the optic nerve lesion) predict future multiphasic disease more strongly, whereas a normal MRI is associated with a lower risk of future activity. In patients who have CIS and a normal cranial MRI, the presence of oligoclonal bands in CSF is sensitive but less specific than MRI for predicting ultimate conversion to CDMS. Nevertheless, using the combination of CSF and MRI findings together does not seem to increase the predictive power significantly over MRI alone, as specified in the McDonald criteria [3,4].

How should this patient be treated?

If a work-up to exclude common alternate causes of demyelination is negative, it is reasonable to monitor the patient without any intervention or, if the symptoms are significantly disabling, to empirically treat with corticosteroids. It is the authors' approach to treat the majority of such patients.

Patient 1 (continued)—a new lesion

The patient's symptoms resolve within 2 weeks. According to the MRI guidelines under the McDonald criteria, dissemination in time can be demonstrated if a new gadolinium-enhancing lesion is seen not less than 3 months after onset of clinical symptoms. Accordingly, she has follow-up MRI of the brain 3 months later, which demonstrates the interval development of a single, ovoid, right-sided periventricular T2 lesion that does not enhance.

Does this patient have clinically definite multiple sclerosis?

Assuming that other causes are excluded, this patient's MRI shows evidence of dissemination in space but does not fulfill the criteria for dissemination in time, as the new lesion on this scan does not enhance. The authors believe, however, that clinicians must consider that enhancement of new inflammatory lesions can be short-lived and, as such, the evolution of a new T2 abnormality likely does constitute temporal dissemination of the disease process. The size of the abnormality may be germane to this thought process. A small (perhaps up to a few millimeters) nonenhancing T2 lesion may have been present on the initial scan but was not identified given the slice protocol. A larger lesion is less likely to be excluded under these circumstances. A very small enhancing lesion at baseline also could be missed yet possibly can be enhancing and identified 3 months later (even though most lesions retain gadolinium for only a few weeks, there are exceptions).

The McDonald criteria are more specific than previous criteria [5], allowing for an earlier diagnosis of CDMS but are criticized for being too stringent (thereby diminishing sensitivity), as illustrated by this case in which CDMS remains undiagnosed despite mounting clinical suspicion with the development of a new brain lesion. A delay in treatment intervention for a patient likely to have multiphasic disease (such as this one) precludes the ability to reduce either the risk of relapse number and severity, the development of new brain or spinal cord lesions, or the progression of neurologic disability. A review by the Therapeutics and Technology Assessment Subcommittee of the American Academy of Neurology, published 2 years after the unveiling of the McDonald criteria, finds that the presence of three or more white matter lesions on baseline T2-weighted MRI in patients who have CIS is a sensitive predictor of conversion to CDMS, especially if lesions are periventricular [6]. The review also finds that new T2 or new enhancing lesions on follow-up imaging are highly predictive of CDMS development if the baseline MRI shows two or more enhancing lesions.

With regard to this particular patient who has CIS and who presented with only a single lesion on MRI at baseline, MS may be kept as a tentative working diagnosis while the patient is monitored for the evolution of either more definitive evidence for multiphasic disease (essentially MS) or the emergence of new information that leads to the confirmation of an alternate cause (not likely, but possible).

Should this patient be started on disease-modifying therapy?

Two prospective, double-blinded, randomized, placebo-controlled trials find that patients who have CIS and abnormal MRIs benefit from interferon-β1a therapy even if they do not completely fulfill the McDonald criteria for CDMS [7,8]. The Controlled High-Risk Subjects Avonex Multiple Sclerosis Prevention Study (CHAMPS) trial (using 30 μg of weekly intramuscular interferon-β1a) finds a lower cumulative probability of developing CDMS, reductions in volume of brain lesions, fewer new or enlarging lesions, and fewer enhancing lesions during the follow-up period, whereas the Early Treatment of Multiple Sclerosis (ETOMS) trial (using weekly subcutaneous interferon-β1a at 22 μg) demonstrates a more prolonged time to conversion to CDMS, a reduction in annualized relapse rates, fewer numbers of new T2 MRI lesions, and a smaller increase in overall lesion burden. The MRI criteria for inclusion into these studies, however, were defined as either two clinically silent lesions at least 3 mm in diameter (for the CHAMPS trial) or three to four white matter lesions (for ETOMS). The benefits demonstrated in these trials cannot be extrapolated directly to this patient's case, as she had only one lesion at baseline. A compelling argument for starting therapy can be made, however, if MS is highly suspected and other diseases have been reasonably excluded.

What other diseases besides multiple sclerosis are in the differential diagnosis?

Because of the absence of any specific confirmatory laboratory test, MS remains a clinical diagnosis that is reliant on the exclusion of other mimicking conditions (Box 1). Laboratory evaluation necessarily is driven by clinical suspicion, which can reasonably exclude many of these conditions based

Box 1. Conditions that mimic multiple sclerosis

Intracranial syndromes
Cerebrovascular disease
Hyperhomocysteinemia
Antiphospholipid antibody syndrome
Cerebral autosomal dominant arteriopathy with subcortical infarcts
    and leukoencephalopathy (CADASIL)
Arterio-venous malformation
Migraine
Susac's
Cogan's
Syphilis
Lyme
Marchiafava-Bignami
Primary CNS vasculitis
Behcet's
HIV
Progressive multifocal leukoencephalopathy (PML)
Osmotic myelinolysis
Reversible posterior leukoencephalopathy
Congenital Leukodystrophy
Mitochondrial disorders
Sarcoidosis
Systemic lupus erythematosus
Sjogren's
Rheumatoid arthritis
Lymphoma
Glioma
Acute disseminated encephalomyelitis

Spinal syndromes
Arterio-venous malformation
Syphilis
Lyme
HIV
Human T-cell lymphotrophic virus type 1
Vertebral spondylarthropathy
Neuromyelitis opticans
Vitamin B_{12} deficiency
Vitamin E deficiency
Nitrous oxide toxicity
Copper deficiency
Zinc toxicity
Spinal cord ischemia

on elements of history, familial or social risk factors, and clinical examination. Nevertheless, the initial work-up usually includes serum testing for inflammatory screening with erythrocyte sedimentation rate, C-reactive protein (CRP), antinuclear antibody, angiotensin-converting enzyme levels, and anti-neutrophil cytoplasmic antibodies (ANCA); infectious screening for syphilis, HIV, and Lyme disease; and metabolic screening for vitamin B_{12} deficiency and thyroid dysfunction.

Patient 2—relapsing remitting multiple sclerosis on disease-modifying therapy with breakthrough relapses

A 39-year-old woman suffers an episode of optic neuritis and is found to have multiple white matter lesions consistent with MS on MRI. A course of intravenous (IV) steroids is given with subsequent recovery of vision after 2 weeks. She is started on thrice-weekly subcutaneous interferon-β1a injections (Rebif) and remains clinically stable until 5 months later when she notices the onset of left leg numbness and dysesthesias. Repeat MRI shows the emergence of a new enhancing lesion in her right parietal subcortical white matter and she receives another course of steroids with resolution of symptoms. She is continued on her disease-modifying therapy and does well until 20 months later when her right hand becomes clumsy while washing dishes. Symptoms do not abate with cooling and rest, and follow-up MRI shows a new enhancing lesion in her left frontal lobe and the interval development of two new, nonenhancing lesions within the right centrum semiovale.

How should this patient be managed?

The initial variable that needs to be evaluated in this patient is noncompliance with the injection medication, which commonly may be because of lack of perceived benefit or development of intolerable dermatologic or systemic side effects [9]. Psychosocial circumstances, such as depression, forgetfulness, and economic difficulty, may be prominent factors that have an impact on therapy adherence.

Interventions that can help improve compliance include reinforcement of realistic patient expectations from disease-modifying therapy, attending to patients' emotional status with regard to depression, fostering a close therapeutic alliance between health care providers and patients, and promoting patients' sense of independence and personal control over their therapy and its potential benefits [10]. Patients should be instructed on techniques for minimizing skin reactions to the disease-modifying agent (DMA) injections, such as allowing the medication to warm up to room temperature; using shorter needle lengths for appropriate patients (eg, those on intramuscular therapy and who have a lean body mass); rotating injection sites; using auto-injectors; applying local anesthestics or ice before injection; maintaining systematic sterile procedures; and using preinjection and postinjection anti-inflammatories, such as long-acting naproxen (Naprelan), or low-dose oral steroids to reduce the systemic flulike side effects of interferons [11,12]. Patients who have postinjection headaches respond well to triptans, such as eletriptan (Relpax).

Recent reports have added significantly to knowledge about the impact of neutralizing antibodies (NABs) on interferons. Up to 41% of all patients on various interferon therapies eventually may develop persistent NABs, usually within the first 12 to 24 months after initiating treatment. Those who remain NAB-free for that time period typically do not need to be re-tested subsequently [13]. The risk of NAB development is substantially higher for patients on interferon-β1b (Betaseron) and subcutaneous interferon-β1a (Rebif) compared with weekly intramuscular interferon-β1a (Avonex) and likely relates to several factors, including drug formulation, dose, frequency, and route of administration. Once patients persistently test positive for NABs, they suffer reduced treatment benefits with respect to relapse rates, Expanded Disability Status Scale (EDSS) progression, and MRI lesion burden compared with those who remain NAB negative [14,15]. Patients who have breakthrough relapses should be tested for NABs at 12 to 18 months after starting therapy, and, if the levels are persistently high, they can be transitioned to either glatiramer acetate or other immune-modifying therapy (eg, pulse intermittent steroids, azathioprine [Imuran], mycophenolate mofetil [Cellcept], and so forth). Some patients who become NAB positive may revert back to NAB-negative status during subsequent months, but the majority remain NAB positive for several years [13].

If patients have no problems with adherence or NABs, then the addition of another medication to the DMA should be considered, as more frequent relapses may accelerate progression of disability. One commonly used option is regularly scheduled pulses of corticosteroids, which are found, in a small, phase II clinical trial to reduce increases in T1 black hole volume, to diminish increases in whole-brain atrophy, and to delay clinical progression during a 5-year follow-up period, even though no effects are found on annualized relapse rate or changes in T2 lesion volume [16]. Protocols for steroid administration are highly variable and can range from monthly pulses (1 g methylprednisolone/d for 1 day) to quarterly pulses (every 3 months) (1 g methylprednisolone/d for 3 consecutive days). Although IV methylprednisolone historically is the preferred formulation, the equivalent oral dose of methylprednisolone, prednisone, or dexamethasone may be used. Preliminary investigations suggest no significant differences between oral and IV corticosteroid formulations in terms of bioavailability [17], gastric tolerance [18], rate of recovery from acute relapses [19], or overall relapse rate in relapsing remitting MS (RRMS) [20]. The exact effect of pulse steroids on the incidence of osteoporosis and subsequent bone fractures is poorly characterized, because bone density also may be affected adversely by other aspects of MS, such as immobility. It is suggested that steroids may only increase the occurrence of osteopenia without significantly affecting the risk of osteoporosis [21]. Nevertheless, the authors routinely screen all patients, young and old, female and male, for diminutions of bone density with dual x-ray absorptiometry and consider the use of calcium, vitamin D, and bisphosphonate supplementation in individual patients.

In addition to adjunctive steroid therapy, other medications that may be considered in combination with injectable DMAs in patients who have breakthrough disease include mitoxantrone (Novantrone), cyclophosphamide (Cytoxan), azathioprine, methotrexate, mycophenolate mofetil, and IV immunoglobulin (IVIg). The authors often consider combining an injectable DMA with a daily immunosuppressant, such as azathioprine or mycophenolate, along with quarterly pulses of steroids (or IVIg when steroids either are ineffective or contraindicated). Alternately, cyclophosphamide is a reasonable first choice in this case, as it can benefit patients who have signs of active inflammation on MRI and who enjoy a low level of disability by EDSS [22,23]. Mitoxantrone can be a highly effective temporizing therapy to reduce inflammation, relapses, and progression but can be associated with cardiotoxicity and risk of leukemia. Patients who have transitioned to a more progressive, neurodegenerative (and less inflammatory phase of the disease) course with infrequent relapses and few enhancing lesions but greater disability may not see as much benefit from mitoxantrone or cyclophosphamide, as these agents seem to exert more of an anti-inflammatory, T-cell mediated effect [24].

There is some evidence from nonblinded trials that methotrexate and azathioprine have beneficial effects on relapse rate and MRI parameters while remaining safe and well tolerated [25–27], but more definitive studies to evaluate the use of these agents in RRMS are lacking. The clinical efficacy of mycophenolate mofetil has yet to demonstrated in clinical trials.

Could this patient be switched from current interferon to another injectable disease-modifying agent?

This is an option to be considered in many patients. The authors find, however, that those who are adherent with their treatment and are NAB negative on interferon therapy often continue to exhibit ongoing disease activity if simply converted from one interferon to another (irrespective of dose and frequency). Despite this, there are subsets of patients who tend to benefit more from one preparation than another and those who respond best to either interferon or glatiramer acetate. As such, converting from one DMA to another is an option available to neurologists who are confronting patients exhibiting breakthrough disease. In the majority of active patients, the authors typically intensify treatment (rather than switch) by coupling a platform DMA with adjunctive therapy (most commonly pulse steroids with azathioprine, methotrexate, or mycophenolate).

Patient 3—relapsing remitting multiple sclerosis transitioning to secondary progressive multiple sclerosis

A 48-year-old man is diagnosed with CDMS after an episode of left-sided optic neuritis and the discovery of multiple white matter lesions on MRI, one of which is enhancing. Vision improves after a course of steroids, but then he is lost to follow-up for 4 years. He returns to the clinic with a 4-day history of right hemiparesis and is found to have more lesions on MRI, with an enhancing lesion in his left frontal lobe. A second course of steroids is followed by initiation of weekly intramuscular interferon-β1a and his right hemiparesis resolves after 3 months of physical therapy. He then is diligent with his follow-up care and remains clinically stable during the next 3 years until his wife reports that he is having difficulty keeping regular employment, being unable to keep up with the pace of work at a succession of fast-food restaurants. He confesses that his concentration seems more impaired and that he is distracted easily. Repeat MRI reveals the interval development of mild ventriculomegaly (consistent with brain atrophy) but otherwise stable lesion load. A careful history does not find evidence for depression or sleep disturbance. There is no evidence of anemia or thyroid dysfunction and his vitamin B_{12} level is normal. His wife confirms that he has been compliant with his DMA and testing for NABs is negative. Neuropsychologic testing finds deficits in concentration, memory, and processing speed consistent with a subcortical process. Over the next 6 months, he continues to have progressive concentration and processing problems, eventually filing for disability because of cognitive impairment. He also develops intermittent urinary incontinence, although his ambulation and motor skills seem intact, and his wife reports that spontaneous conversation and activity level have declined such that he spends much of his time watching TV.

How should this patient be managed?

This patient is transitioning from RRMS to secondary progressive MS (SPMS) without overt clinical relapses despite interferon treatment. His disease progression involves primarily cognitive decline, which may have a minimal impact on his EDSS score. The therapeutic option at this point is mitoxantrone, an anthracenedione used to treat certain neoplasms, which is the only FDA-approved agent for SPMS, worsenng RRMS, and progressive-relapsing MS. The usefulness of this medication is limited, however, by its adverse effects [28]. This includes a dose-dependent myocardial toxicity that can lead to irreversible heart failure, such that mitoxantrone can be administered only up to a cumulative lifetime dose of 140 mg/m^2. Because usually it is given in increments of 12 mg/m^2 every 3 months, this allows a duration of therapy of only 2 to 3 years. A dose-related increase in the risk of leukemia also is observed in cancer patients treated with mitoxantrone; in the MS population, this is limited to a small number of case reports but remains a serious consideration. As the benefit of mitoxantrone on arresting disease progression can be somewhat modest, the risk-benefit ratio in individual cases must be considered carefully before it is administered.

Another option for this patient is pulse cyclophosphamide therapy, which is the subject of many clinical trials evaluating its use in progressive MS. The results of these studies are conflicting, with earlier trials finding no significant benefit [29,30] in contrast to more recent findings suggesting that the agent may be more useful in certain subtypes of patients who have progressive MS than in others, such as those who have a shorter duration of progression before treatment, those who have relapses in addition to progression during the 2 years before therapy, and patients of a younger age [24,31,32]. With regard to this particular case, there also is evidence that cyclophosphamide in combination with methylprednisolone improves cognitive function in patients who have progressive MS [33]. There are several adverse effects associated with cyclophosphamide, most commonly involving alopecia, gastrointestinal upset, infection, hemorrhagic cystitis, infertility, and a risk of secondary neoplasms with cumulative doses greater than 80 g, but this side effect profile is easier to manage in comparison to that of mitoxantrone. The allowable duration of therapy also is much longer than that of mitoxantrone.

Another option that the authors consider with progression to SPMS include pulse steroids with or without the use of daily or weekly immunosuppression, such as with azathioprine, mycophenolate, and methotrexate. A recent trial finds that IVIg is not beneficial in patients who have SPMS [34].

Patient 4—symptomatic therapy

A 49-year-old woman with a diagnosis of SPMS has moved into the area from another city and presents to a clinic for establishment of neurologic care. Her disease course is characterized by right optic neuritis at 23 years of age followed a few years later by an episode of left hemiparesis. Both events resolved without residual deficits. She has multiple MRI lesions characteristic of demyelination disseminated throughout her brain and spinal cord. Ten years ago, she was started on interferon-β1b therapy and always has tested negative for NABs. She has had slowly progressive spastic paraparesis for the past 8 years but still is able to ambulate with the aid of a single-prong cane. Her main concern currently is persistent fatigue, which she describes as "draining." Her fatigue is exacerbated at times by heat, most recently while traversing the parking lot from her car to the clinic under the hot summer sun, but she also is plagued by a persistent "lack of energy" that initially responded to modafinil (Provigil) but has recurred despite daily compliance with the medication. Under further questioning, she concedes to sleeping somewhat poorly but has done so for "a long time" and does suffer from symptoms of excessive daytime sleepiness. She usually awakens once or twice per night with the urge to urinate but frequently does not void or has small urinary volumes with a feeling of incomplete emptying. Additionally, she suffers from occasional leg spasms that sometimes arouse her briefly during the night and resolve after a few minutes. Pertinent findings on examination reveal increased tone in her legs, right more so than left, and circumduction of the right leg during the 25-foot timed walking test, which is recorded at 18 seconds. Her muscle tone is relieved modestly with baclofen (Lioresal) but she feels that the stiffness in her legs objectively has worsened over the previous 6 months. She becomes somewhat tearful after the walking test and, after careful probing by the clinician, reluctantly admits to feeling helpless, frustrated, and depressed. She is preoccupied with her ongoing neurologic deterioration. Toward the end of the visit, the patient mentions in passing that she recently has been suffering spontaneous episodes of brief shooting pains involving her left ear that are becoming bothersome.

How should this patient be managed?

The complexity of symptoms illustrated in this vignette is a common theme in patients who have MS and busy clinicians easily may feel overwhelmed amid tight clinic schedules. Of note, other frequently encountered MS-related symptom complexes are not dealt with in this case, such as bowel and sexual dysfunction, bone demineralization, assistive devices, and cognitive decline. The authors' experience is that addressing these issues in a thorough and systematic fashion during office visits tends to optimize the global interdisciplinary management of patients who have MS, reduce follow-up telephone calls, decrease noncompliance issues, and minimize difficulties in physician-patient relationships that can strain clinic resources.

In approaching this patient's main concern of fatigue, it is essential to consider secondary causes, such as hypothyroidism, anemia, liver or kidney dysfunction, cardiopulmonary disease, underlying infection, chronic pain, and sleep disorders, such as obstructive sleep apnea. Although fatigue is a well-known cardinal symptom of MS itself, some of these comorbid conditions are common and should be treated accordingly. In this case, possible contributing factors to the patient's fatigue are mood disturbance, heat sensitivity, sleep interruption from her nocturia and muscle spasms, increased work requirement of walking derived from her worsening spasticity, and primary MS-related fatigue. She also seems to suffer from episodes of neuropathic pain, which can contribute to feelings of fatigue and mental exhaustion if persistent or severe. Although a more comprehensive review of symptom management is beyond the scope of this article, an approach to each of these problems is discussed briefly.

The patient's urinary symptoms are consistent with detrusor sphincter dyssynergia, where damage to spinal cord tracts results in a loss of coordination between detrusor muscle contraction and sphincter relaxation, leading to feelings of urgency with urinary retention as the bladder wall spasms against a closed outflow tract. The authors find that certain behavioral modifications, such as limiting fluid intake in the early evening before bedtime and scheduled voiding every 3 to 4 hours during the day, can help reduce bladder expansion and reduce feelings of urgency in certain patients. Patients also are counseled to avoid caffeine and spicy foods containing capsaicin that can irritate the bladder wall and induce detrusor spasms. Pharmaceutical options for detrusor sphincter dyssynergia include anticholinergics, such as oxybutynin (Ditropan), tolterodine (Detrol), solifenacin (Vesicare), and trospium (Sanctura), which act to reduce detrusor contraction. These medications may be limited by ineffectiveness or side effects, such as gastric retention, drowsiness, or dry mouth. To promote sphincteric relaxation and more complete emptying, an α-adrenergic antagonist, such as tamsulosin (Flomax), can be used effectively in many patients and potentially avoid the requirement for clean intermittent catheterization.

With regard to this patient's muscle tone, it again is important to consider and treat secondary triggers for increases in tone, such as pain, dehydration, constipation, infection, fatigue, restless legs syndrome, and even deep venous thrombosis. It also is helpful to distinguish between phasic increases in tone, which are exemplified here by nocturnal leg cramps, and tonic increases in tone, such as the spasticity, which affect her walking. The authors' experience has shown that clonazepam (Klonopin) is quite effective in paroxysmal muscle spasms, but that other agents such as diazepam (Valium), gabapentin (Neurontin), tizanidine (Zanaflex), quinine sulfate, and dopamine agonists, can also be useful. Tonic increases in tone are best addressed initially with a combination of physical therapy and home stretching exercises. If spasticity progresses in spite of these remedies, then medications such as baclofen, tizanidine, clonazepam, or even levetiracetam (Keppra) can be used either alone or in combination. Intrathecal baclofen pumps are useful in carefully selected patients who have baclofen-responsive spasticity but a low threshold for adverse effects or are increasingly recalcitrant to oral agents.

Mood disturbances are prevalent in the MS population, but patients may not volunteer symptoms of anxiety or depression during clinic visits. Given the variety and efficacy of interventions available to treat disorders of mood, it is incumbent on the clinician to ask patients about these symptoms. A social support network of friends, family, and financial resources is crucial in maintaining emotional well being, so the authors inquire routinely about interpersonal relationships and other sources of psychosocial stress during clinic visits, often enlisting the aid of counseling psychologists and social workers for help in resolving emotional and financial conflicts. The authors also prescribe antidepressants, such as venlafaxine (Effexor), bupropion (Wellbutrin), and escitalopram (Lexapro), or other selective serotonin reuptake inhibitors, which are useful but more effective if psychosocial factors are addressed adequately.

Neuropathic pain frequently is encountered in MS, with trigeminal neuralgia a well-known example; this patient may have geniculate neuralgia, a less common variety. The agents that the authors find useful include anticonvulsants, such as phenytoin (Dilantin), carbamazepine (Tegretol), oxcarbazepine (Trileptal), lamotrigine (Lamictal), gabapentin, and levetiracetam; antidepressants, such as tricyclics and duloxetine (Cymbalta); and topical compounded formulations of lidocaine, gabapentin, dextromethorphan, amitriptyline, and baclofen. More recently, the authors find that direct injections of botulinum toxin can mitigate neuropathic pain significantly.

Not surprisingly, with chronic pain conditions, it is difficult to predict which will be the single most effective agent for any given patient. Individual medications need to be administered for a sufficient period of time and at an appropriate dose (often requiring significant escalation) before the full value of treatment can be determined.

Primary MS-related fatigue is diagnosed when all other secondary causes of fatigue are excluded or treated adequately. Perhaps more than any other, this symptom may limit patient activities significantly, even in the absence of any focal neurologic debilitation. Among the medications available to treat MS-related fatigue, the authors find that modafinil (Provigil) is effective and convenient to use. Patients in the authors' clinic are started on initial daily doses of 25 mg and titrated up to 200 mg as necessary. The authors also find that many patients do not require the medication every day to alleviate their fatigue and can be dosed on an as-needed basis. Other medications that can be useful if modafinil fails to give benefit include amantadine (Symmetrel), methylphenidate (Ritalin or Concerta), and extended-release amphetamine/dextroamphetamine (Adderall XR).

Heat sensitivity is a well-known phenomenon in MS and occasionally can be life threatening, such as an Uhthoff's-related weakness induced by submergence in a hot water whirlpool or bathtub that leads to drowning. Patients who find that their fatigue is exacerbated significantly by heat may feel better after liberal consumption of ice-cold beverages, in particular those made from crushed or shaved ice, and personal cooling systems available from sports shops and internet vendors that consist of articles of clothing that use miniature fans, ice packs, or phase-change gels to maintain a lower body surface temperature. In terms of medication, 4-aminopyridine is a potassium channel-blocking agent used for many years to treat a variety of symptoms in patients who have MS and can be beneficial in up to two thirds of patients who have heat-sensitive fatigue. It currently can be obtained only from compounding pharmacies and needs to be taken with food and kept in dark storage. The authors start patients on 5-mg morning doses, which can be increased every few days up to 10 mg 3 times a day. The authors' experience is that limiting patients to no more than 10 mg per dose minimizes the dose-dependent risk of seizure .

Frequently, patients report that their fatigue has returned despite daily compliance with a medication; usually this occurs in patients who have had incomplete resolution of their symptoms and feel frustrated that they are not back to their baseline energy level. In these cases, the authors recommend having patients incorporate a 1- or 2-day "drug holiday" once a week, when they suspend taking their antifatigue medicine for an entire day. This has the effect of allowing them to feel the return of their fatigue to the nadir, whereupon they appreciate the significant benefit of the agent despite its inability to eradicate their fatigue fully. This does not increase the efficacy of the medication so much as change the patient point of reference and perception of treatment benefit.

Summary

Although substantial capabilities have emerged in the ability to globally manage patients who have MS, clinicians continue to be confronted with formidable challenges. Reduction in disease activity and its impact on disability progression remains the central objective of disease-modifying therapy and most current MS research initiatives. Nevertheless, the principal factors that determine the day-to-day limitations on functional capabilities (activities of daily living, work performance, quality of life, and so forth) are a derivative of the pathophysiology of the disease process itself. The substrate for these limitations is inherent in the pathology of demyelination and axonal dysfunction. Identifying measures that can optimize the performance and fidelity of axonal conduction mechanisms may translate into a reduction in MS-related symptoms. Chronic neurologic disease management (with MS representing a signature example) can be optimized when all members of the care team (including patients and their families) collaborate in the coordination of interdisciplinary care models that address all aspects of suffering.

References

[1] McDonald WI, Compston A, Edan G, et al. Recommended diagnostic criteria for multiple sclerosis: guidelines from the International Panel on the Diagnosis of Multiple Aclerosis. Ann Neurol 2001;50:121–7.
[2] Beck RW, Trobe JD, Moke PS, et al. High- and low-risk profiles for the development of multiple sclerosis within 10 years after optic neuritis. Arch Ophthalmol 2003;121:944–9.
[3] Tintore M, Rovira A, Brieva L, et al. Isolated demyelinating syndromes: comparison of CSF oligoclonal bands and different MR imaging criteria to predict conversion to CDMS. Mult Scler 2001;7:359–63.

[4] Sastre-Garriga J, Tintore M, Rovira A, et al. Conversion to multiple sclerosis after a clinically isolated syndrome of the brainstem: cranial magnetic resonance imaging, cerebrospinal fluid and neurophysiological findings. Mult Scler 2003;9:39–43.

[5] Barkhof F, Filippi M, Miller DH, et al. Comparison of MRI criteria at first presentation to predict conversion to clinically definite multiple sclerosis. Brain 1997;120(Pt 11): 2059–69.

[6] Frohman EM, Goodin DS, Calabresi PA, et al. The utility of MRI in suspected MS: report of the Therapeutics and Technology Assessment Subcommittee of the American Academy of Neurology. Neurology 2003;61:602–11.

[7] Jacobs LD, Beck RW, Simon JH, et al. Intramuscular interferon beta-1a therapy initiated during a first demyelinating event in multiple sclerosis. N Engl J Med 2000;343: 898–904.

[8] Comi G, Filippi M, Barkhof F, et al. Effect of early interferon treatment on conversion to definite multiple sclerosis: a randomised study. Lancet 2001;357:1576–82.

[9] Ruggieri RM, Settipani N, Viviano L, et al. Long-term interferon-beta treatment for multiple sclerosis. Neurol Sci 2003;24:361–4.

[10] Mohr DC, Goodkin DE, Masuoka L, et al. Treatment adherence and patient retention in the first year of a Phase-III clinical trial for the treatment of multiple sclerosis. Mult Scler 1999;5: 192–7.

[11] Frohman EM, Brannon K, Alexander S, et al. Disease modifying agent related skin reactions in multiple sclerosis: prevention, assessment, and management. Mult Scler 2004;10:302–7.

[12] Frohmann E, Phillips T, Kokel K, et al. Disease-modifying therapy in multiple sclerosis: strategies for optimizing management. Neurologist 2002;8:227–36.

[13] Sorensen PS, Koch-Henriksen N, Ross C, et al. Appearance and disappearance of neutralizing antibodies during interferon-beta therapy. Neurology 2005;65:33–9.

[14] Francis GS, Rice GPA, Alsop JC; PRISMS Study Group. Interferon beta-1a in MS: results following development of neutralizing antibodies in PRISMS. Neurology 2005;65:48–55.

[15] Kappos L, Clanet M, Sandberg-Wollheim M, et al. Neutralizing antibodies and efficacy of interferon beta-1a: a 4-year controlled study. Neurology 2005;65:40–7.

[16] Zivadinov R, Rudick RA, De Masi R, et al. Effects of IV methylprednisolone on brain atrophy in relapsing-remitting MS. Neurology 2001;57:1239–47.

[17] Morrow SA, Stoian CA, Dmitrovic J, et al. The bioavailability of IV methylprednisolone and oral prednisone in multiple sclerosis. Neurology 2004;63:1079–80.

[18] Metz LM, Sabuda D, Hilsden RJ, et al. Gastric tolerance of high-dose pulse oral prednisone in multiple sclerosis. Neurology 1999;53:2093–6.

[19] Barnes D, Hughes RAC, Morris RW, et al. Randomised trial of oral and intravenous methylprednisolone in acute relapses of multiple sclerosis. Lancet 1997;349:902–6.

[20] Sharrack B, Hughes RAC, Morris RW, et al. The effect of oral and intravenous methylprednisolone treatment on subsequent relapse rate in multiple sclerosis. J Neurol Sci 2000;173: 73–7.

[21] Zorzon M, Zivadinov R, Locatelli L, et al. Long-term effects of intravenous high dose methylprednisolone pulses on bone mineral density in patients with multiple sclerosis. Eur J Neurol 2005;12:550–6.

[22] Reggio E, Nicoletti A, Fiorilla T, et al. The combination of cyclophosphamide plus interferon beta as rescue therapy could be used to treat relapsing-remitting multiple sclerosis patients. Twenty-four months follow-up. J Neurol 2005;252:1255–61.

[23] Smith D. Preliminary analysis of a trial of pulse cyclophosphamide in IFN-beta-resistant active MS. J Neurol Sci 2004;223:73–9.

[24] Weiner HL, Cohen JA. Treatment of multiple sclerosis with cyclophosphamide: critical review of clinical and immunologic effects. Mult Scler 2002;8:142–54.

[25] Cavazzuti M, Merelli E, Tassone G, et al. Lesion load quantification in serial MR of early relapsing multiple sclerosis patients in azathioprine treatment. A retrospective study. Eur Neurol 1997;38:284–90.

[26] Lus G, Romano F, Scuotto A, et al. Azathioprine and interferon beta(1a) in relapsing-remitting multiple sclerosis patients: increasing efficacy of combined treatment. Eur Neurol 2004;
51:15–20.

[27] Calabresi PA, Wilterdink JL, Rogg JM, et al. An open-label trial of combination therapy
with interferon beta-1a and oral methotrexate in MS. Neurology 2002;58:314–7.

[28] Goodin DS, Anason BG, Coyle PK, et al. The use of mitoxantrone (Novantrone) for the
treatment of multiple sclerosis. Report of the Therapeutics and Technology Assessment Subcommittee of the American Academy of Neurology. Neurology 2003;61:1332–8.

[29] Likosky WH, Fireman B, Elmore R, et al. Intense immunosuppression in chronic progressive multiple sclerosis: the Kaiser study. J Neurol Neurosurg Psychiatry 1991;54:1055–60.

[30] The Canadian Cooperative Multiple Sclerosis Study Group. The Canadian cooperative trial
of cyclophosphamide and plasma exchange in progressive multiple sclerosis. Lancet 1991;
337:441–6.

[31] Hohol MJ, Olek MJ, Orave EJ, et al. Treatment of progressive multiple sclerosis with pulse
cyclophosphamide/methylprednisolone: response to therapy is linked to the duration of progressive disease. Mult Scler 1999;5:403–9.

[32] Weiner HL, Mackin GA, Orave EJ, et al. Intermittent cyclophosphamide pulse therapy in
progressive multiple sclerosis: final report of the Northeast Cooperative Multiple Sclerosis
Treatment Group. Neurology 1993;43:910–8.

[33] Zephir H, de Seze J, Duhardin K, et al. One-year cyclophosphamide treatment combined
with methylprednisolone improves cognitive dysfunction in progressive forms of multiple
sclerosis. Mult Scler 2005;11:360–3.

[34] Hommes OR, Sorensen PS, Fazekas F, et al. Intravenous immunoglobulin in secondary progressive multiple sclerosis: randomised placebo-controlled trial. Lancet 2004;364:1149–56.

ELSEVIER
SAUNDERS

Neurol Clin 24 (2006) 215–231

NEUROLOGIC
CLINICS

Syncope: Case Studies

Ronald Schondorf, PhD, MD[a],*, Win-Kuang Shen, MD[b]

[a]*Department of Neurology, Sir Mortimer B. Davis Jewish General Hospital,
McGill University, 3755 Chemin de la Cote Ste Catherine, Montreal,
Quebec H3T 1E2, Canada*
[b]*Department of Cardiology, Mayo Clinic, Rochester, MN 55905, USA*

Neurologists are often called upon to diagnose the cause of self-limited transient loss of consciousness without associated concussion, which essentially means distinguishing syncope from seizure [1]. To diagnose syncope one must be reasonably sure that the transient loss of consciousness is due to transient global cerebral hypoperfusion [2]. As the patient is often perfectly well at the time of examination, one is left mainly with the clinical history and occasionally with the physical examination to help make this determination. Tests that delineate the etiology of syncope are useful when a direct correlation can be made between event and abnormality. In most cases, however, the etiology of syncope is at best presumptive because an abnormality is discovered independent of syncope or when a false-positive provocation of syncope occurs. In this article, the authors present a series of patient vignettes that highlight the salient clinical features of various conditions that cause transient global cerebral hypoperfusion. Relevant testing modalities and treatments are also discussed.

Case 1: syncope in a young woman with a normal exam

A 22-year-old right-handed woman was referred for two episodes of loss of consciousness. The first episode occurred 4 months before consultation. The previous night the patient had consumed some wine but not to excess. The following morning she awoke with unexplained malaise and lost consciousness while in the bathroom. She lacerated her chin and required sutures. Routine blood chemistry, complete blood count (CBC), and electrocardiogram (ECG) were normal. Approximately 6 weeks later the

---

* Corresponding author.
E-mail address: ronald.schondorf@mcgill.ca (R. Schondorf).

0733-8619/06/$ - see front matter © 2006 Elsevier Inc. All rights reserved.
doi:10.1016/j.ncl.2006.02.002

patient experienced a second episode of loss of consciousness while standing, this time preceded by premonitory symptoms of warmth and malaise. The duration of loss of consciousness was less than 1 minute and there was no postictal confusion. A witness noticed some trembling during the episode but no obvious jerking movements. There was no tongue biting or urinary incontinence. There was no history of orthostatic intolerance; however, the patient had a history of febrile convulsions as a child, and a maternal uncle had epilepsy. Neurologic examination was normal, and there was no postural drop in blood pressure. A CT scan and an electroencephalogram (EEG) requested by another physician were normal. After discussion with the patient, an 80° head-up tilt table test was performed for reassurance and for patient education. The results of this test are shown in Fig. 1. A diagnosis of benign vasovagal syncope was made, and therapeutic options were discussed.

Can the diagnosis be made on clinical grounds alone?

The diagnosis of vasovagal syncope is suggested by loss of consciousness precipitated by prolonged standing or stressful stimuli (fear, pain, invasive instrumentation). Common associated stressors include increased ambient or body core temperature, lack of food, and rapid early morning rising [3]. Typical prodromal features include lightheadedness, fatigue, blurred vision, sweating, nausea, and palpitations [3]. Similar premonitory symptoms are also seen in patients with cardiac syncope, but the absence of

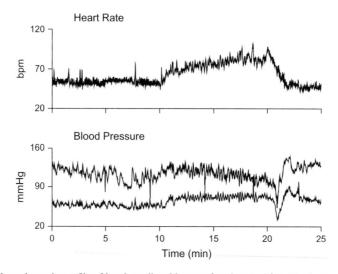

Fig. 1. Hemodynamic profile of head-up tilt-table test of patient 1. After 10 minutes of supine rest, the patient was tilted. The increase in heart rate is appropriate, and there is a mild tachycardia at syncope (minute 21) where a rapid collapse in systolic and diastolic blood pressure is noted.

significant cardiac disease makes the diagnosis of vasovagal syncope much more likely. The clinical exam of patients with vasovagal syncope is often normal, although in some cases a transient (less than 30 seconds) drop in blood pressure can be detected upon rapid standing from the supine or squat position. Vasovagal syncope may often occur in clusters and may then not recur for months to years. A history of syncope in childhood or in related family members may suggest vasovagal syncope in young adults [4, 5]. However, the neurologist should be aware of the existence of unique groups of patients with primary rhythm disorders in the absence of any structural heart disease who may present with syncope without any cardiac abnormalities on examination. A family history of syncope and sudden cardiac death should alert the neurologist to this possibility, and a 12-lead ECG should always be performed.

The presence of palpitations before loss of consciousness [6] or lack of premonitory nausea may be more commonly seen in cardiogenic than noncardiogenic syncope [7]. It is critical to distinguish between these two classes of syncope because patients with cardiac syncope have higher mortality rates compared with those of noncardiac or unknown causes. Syncope of cardiac cause does not confer additional mortality risk when compared with nonsyncopal patients with similar degrees of heart disease [8], but a cardiac cause of syncope often suggests previously unsuspected cardiac disease. Should syncope occur in a patient with evidence of underlying structural cardiac disease, the probability of cardiogenic syncope is significantly higher than in a patient without evidence of cardiac disease. In the absence of structural heart disease, cardiogenic syncope should be suspected if there is a history of bifascicular block, asystole, supraventricular tachycardia, or diabetes [9]. A history of blue color noted by bystanders as well as syncope that started above the age of 35 may also suggest that syncope is not vasovagal [9].

A recent study has helped define historical criteria that distinguish syncope (cardiac or not) from seizure with a high degree of reliability [10]. Seizure patients were more likely to have cut tongue, bedwetting, déjà vu, mood changes, and hallucinations or trembling before loss of consciousness. During or after loss of consciousness these patients had postictal confusion, muscle pain, headaches, convulsive movements, head turning, unresponsiveness, and blue skin. High numbers of loss of consciousness were also more typical of seizures. Those with syncope had loss of consciousness or presyncope after prolonged sitting or standing, needles, warm environments, and exercise. Before a spell, patients with syncope were more likely to have symptoms of diaphoresis, dyspnea, chest pain, palpitations, warmth, and nausea.

Based on the above considerations—namely, appropriate premonitory symptoms, presence of an orthostatic stress, short duration of loss of consciousness with prompt recovery, absence of cardiac disease, and normal ECG—the diagnosis of vasovagal syncope can be made on clinical criteria alone.

Should tilt-table testing be performed?

Vasovagal syncope may often be elicited in asymptomatic patients by any maneuver that significantly increases venous pooling in the lower extremities [11]. Lesser degrees of venous pooling achieved by 30 to 60 minutes of head-up tilt with foot-rest support elicits syncope in approximately 30% to 50% of patients with recurrent vasovagal syncope but also in about 10% of healthy volunteers. In many instances, head-up tilt is combined with infusion of isoproterenol (1–3 µg/min) or the sublingual administration of nitroglycerin spray (400 µg) [2]. Both protocols seem equivalent in their capacity to increase the sensitivity of the tilt table test to about 70%. Unfortunately, both protocols decrease the test specificity, causing many normal individuals to faint [12]. Invasive instrumentation alone may also increase the likelihood of syncope in normal individuals. Individuals with blood or injury phobia who have no history of syncope during orthostatic stress often faint during tilt-table testing.

Guidelines and indications for tilt-table testing have been published [13]. It is generally agreed that tilt-table testing should be performed in cases of unexplained single episodes of syncope in high-risk settings (potential risk for serious physical injury) or recurrent episodes in the absence of cardiac disease. For the patient in this case study, the authors used tilt-table testing to provide additional reassurance and education regarding premonitory symptoms of impending syncope. Many patients welcome this additional information and request it even when the physician is fully confident of the diagnosis of vasovagal syncope. The recurrence of syncope is often significantly diminished and frequently eliminated once simple reassurance and education is provided.

Therapeutic options for the treatment of vasovagal syncope

As noted previously, the most important aspect of treatment of vasovagal syncope is patient education with clear explanation of the pathophysiology as well as of the benign nature of this condition. Even without detailed education, approximately 75 percent of untreated patients remain syncope free 2 years after undergoing head-up tilt-table testing. Initial advice should include early recognition of warning symptoms and avoidance of triggering events. If triggers cannot be avoided, simple physical counter maneuvers, such as leg crossing, squatting, or placing one foot on a chair, should be used to increase venous return. These maneuvers are effective in aborting syncope induced by head-up tilt [14]. Acute oral ingestion of 16 oz (slightly less than 500 cc) of water is also effective and increases blood pressure by 20 to 30 mmHg within several minutes with the effect sustained for as long as 1 hour. If not contraindicated, the authors suggest that patients increase fluid (2–2.5 L/day) and salt (10 gm) intake and also attempt to improve orthostatic tolerance by improving aerobic fitness. Using this strategy, most patients remain symptom free.

Pharmacologic treatment of vasovagal syncope may be considered for those patients with recurrent syncope that is refractory to standard conservative treatment. There is as yet no conclusive pharmacologic treatment for vasovagal syncope, although several strategies have been attempted [15]. Beta-adrenergic blockade has been used to diminish cardiac contractility and block the direct adrenergic activation of unmyelinated cardiovagal afferents that have been thought to trigger syncope. Disopyramide has been used to achieve this purpose as well as for its anticholinergic blocking of vagally mediated bradycardia. Propantheline has also been used as a vagolytic agent. Other medications, such as methylphenidate, ephedrine, etilefrine, and midodrine, have been used to supplement sympathetic vasoconstrictor activity. Salt loading or fludrocortisone have been used to increase plasma volume. Most treatment strategies, when reported as case series, show a good deal of promise as effective agents, but when subjected to more rigorous testing are generally no more effective than placebo [16,17].

The placebo effect of treatment of vasovagal syncope is clearly important. The North American Vasovagal Pacemaker Study demonstrated overwhelming efficacy of pacemaker insertion as compared with standard pharmacologic treatment in patients with refractory vasovagal syncope [18]. However, when all patients received pacemakers but were blinded as to whether the pacemaker was functioning, there was no benefit to active pacing over the placebo effect of pacemaker insertion [19]. Given that pacing should have no effect on the vasodepressor component of syncope, pacemakers (using a rate drop algorithm) should only be considered in patients with convincing evidence of primary cardioinhibitory vasovagal syncope.

The authors occasionally use midodrine for short-term treatment of syncope associated with significant orthostatic intolerance [20]. A single, randomized double-blind placebo-controlled trial has also demonstrated surprising efficacy of paroxetine as a treatment for vasovagal syncope [21], but because the mechanism of action of this agent in vasovagal syncope is unknown and because of the risks associated with long-term use of this medication, this treatment is not recommended until additional trials are performed [2].

Case 2: situational syncope

A 58-year-old man with a history of mild treated hypertension was referred for recurrent episodes of lightheadedness and near syncope after drinking cold carbonated beverages. Detailed review of systems for symptoms of autonomic dysfunction or syncope was negative. Blood pressure was 140/80 mmHg taken from both arms in the seated position. Similar values were obtained in the supine position, and there was no evidence of a postural decrease in blood pressure. Neurologic examination was normal. Routine ECG, head-up tilt testing, response to the Valsalva maneuver, and carotid sinus massage performed in the supine and upright positions were all normal.

What additional tests should be performed?

The history is entirely compatible with swallow syncope, one of the situational syncopes. Others within the class of reflexly mediated syncopes include micturition, defecation, or cough syncope. Syncopes that are more associated with impeded venous return include syncope after weight lifting or brass instrument playing, although this may also be a significant contributing mechanism to cough syncope. Postexercise syncope may occasionally be a manifestation of a reflexly mediated situational syncope or of early autonomic failure, whereas syncope during actual exercise is more suggestive of cardiac arrhythmia, structural heart disease, or outflow obstruction. Given the implications of missing a serious cardiac abnormality, the authors advocate comprehensive cardiac testing in all cases of postexercise syncope to rule out the conditions listed. Once these have been ruled out, patients can be tested with postexercise hypotension with supine bicycle exercise and continuous blood pressure recordings. Similarly, the response of this patient to the offending stimulus should be tested to better define the nature of the process. As shown in Fig. 2, drinking cold carbonated soda induced a significant sinus pause of 3.2 seconds. There was an associated reduction in blood pressure. Cold beverages without carbonation were unable to provoke this response, highlighting the uniqueness of each stimulus in provoking the swallow syncope. The neural circuitry that mediates this response has yet to be defined. Treatment of this condition depends solely on avoidance of the offending stimulus and reassurance as to the benign nature of the process.

Case 3: recurrent syncope in the elderly

An 82-year-old patient experienced syncope while sitting in the doctor's office. After initial symptoms of lightheadedness while seated, he stood to drink some water and lost consciousness after drinking as he was returning to his chair. The patient was unconscious for less than 1 minute, and the

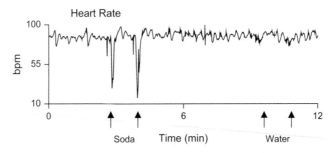

Fig. 2. Transient bradycardia evident during ingestion of cold carbonated beverages, but not cold water, demonstrating selectivity of the stimulus that provokes swallow syncope.

desk attendant was able to feel his pulse as the patient regained consciousness. Within the previous 3 years, the patient has had approximately six
episodes of syncope while sitting, standing, driving, or urinating, usually associated with symptoms of lightheadedness. There was a long-standing history of mild lightheadedness upon standing. The patient had hypertension
treated with a beta blocker but no evidence of coronary artery disease or
other cardiac conditions.

On examination, his heart rate was 65 beats per minute and regular.
Blood pressures were 145/85 mmHg and 110/80 mmHg in the sitting and upright positions, respectively, with mild lightheadedness during stand. Cardiac examination showed a II/VI systolic ejection murmur at the aortic
root. Routine blood work and cardiac enzymes were normal. A 12-lead
ECG showed a PR interval of 220 ms and nonspecific T-wave inversion
in leads II and III. An echocardiogram showed preserved left ventricular
function and mild generalized concentric hypertrophy. There was aortic
sclerosis without stenosis.

Carotid sinus massage performed in the supine position was normal. In
the upright position, left carotid sinus massage induced a 5.3-second pause
(Fig. 3) with complete loss of consciousness. Consciousness was regained
after returning to the supine position. Upon questioning, the patient

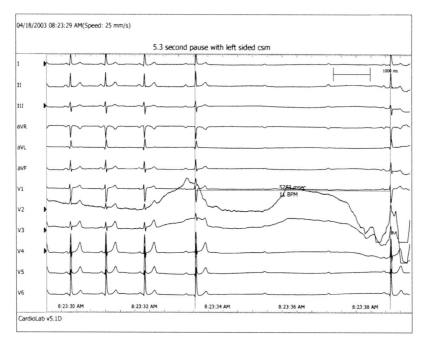

Fig. 3. Rhythm strips from multiple-surface lead channels are shown. During left carotid sinus
massage in the upright position, a 7.8-second pause was induced. This was associated with
syncope.

reported that this was similar to some of his spells, although most of his clinical spells were associated with longer periods of warning. Tilt-table testing was done. Baseline heart rate was 57 beats per minute, and blood pressure was 125/80 mmHg. Immediately upon tilting, heart rate was 65 beats per minute and blood pressure was 120/80 mmHg without any symptoms. At 8 minutes into tilt-table testing, the patient began to experience lightheadedness and diaphoresis. His heart rate slowed to 45 beats per minute, and systolic pressure was in the 70s. He reported that these symptoms were similar to his clinical spells.

Given the presence of significant bradycardia during carotid sinus massage, implantation of a dual-chamber pacemaker was proposed, but the patient was cautioned that this therapy may not completely eliminate symptoms of orthostatic intolerance. The patient has been followed routinely at the outpatient pacemaker clinic for 2 years. The pacemaker function has been normal and there have been no further episodes of syncope, although he has continued to experience some lightheadedness.

Has the correct cause of syncope been diagnosed?

This case highlights the diagnostic challenges that face the physician who diagnoses syncope in the elderly. Syncope is a common cause of falls, injuries, and hospitalizations in older adults as normal age-related physiologic changes often combine with pathologic mechanisms to impair cerebral perfusion. Elderly community-dwelling patients have an average of 3.5 chronic illnesses, as well as receive three times as many medications as the general population. The age-dependent changes, in combination with comorbid medical illnesses, increase the propensity for multiple potential etiologies of syncope in elderly patients. In turn, multiple-cause syncope is an independent predictor of poor clinical outcome [22]. In the case presented, carotid sinus hypersensitivity, vasovagal syncope, and an increased propensity for orthostatic intolerance were found during evaluation. Although one may expect that pacemaker therapy would be effective in treating carotid sinus hypersensitivity and intermittent bradycardia, it would be unlikely that all symptoms related to orthostatic intolerance could be completely eliminated.

Although the diagnostic approach to syncope is not age dependent, it is important to recognize that cardiogenic causes of syncope are more common in the elderly and should be vigorously sought after in this age group through use of noninvasive tests, such as ECG and Holter monitoring. Those with unexplained syncope and an increased risk of a cardiogenic cause may require more detailed cardiac electrophysiology testing or an implantable loop monitor (see below). The patient presented in the case example did not have any significant cardiac abnormalities by history, examination, or ECG, and appropriate abnormalities that mimicked symptoms were obtained during tilt-table testing and carotid sinus massage.

Therefore, more invasive diagnostic studies, such as coronary angiography or electrophysiology study, were not indicated [23,24].

Carotid sinus massage should be a routine part of the examination in elderly patients presenting with syncope unless there is a carotid bruit or history of stroke [2]. This technique is best performed in the upright position by firmly massaging the anterior aspect of the sternocleidomastoid muscle at the level of the cricoid cartilage for 5 to 10 seconds. The response to carotid sinus massage is classified as cardioinhibitory (asystole greater than 3 seconds), vasodepressor (decline in blood pressure greater than 50 mmHg), or mixed, although the reproducibility of these exaggerated cardiovascular responses may vary significantly in a given patient. Continuous noninvasive blood pressure monitoring is required to appreciate the transient vasodepressor component, and the mixed nature of the response can only be appreciated once the cardioinhibitory component of the response is eliminated by atropine or pacing. Patients with a predominantly cardioinhibitory component should be considered for pacemaker insertion but should be cautioned about the possible accompanying vasodepressor component of the response [2].

Case 4: syncope and intermittent bradycardia

A 43-year-old otherwise-healthy man was referred for evaluation of recurrent syncope. Two years prior he had his first episode while seated at a meeting. A brief moment of nausea immediately preceded the loss of consciousness and urinary incontinence. There was no postictal confusion. Neurologic evaluation, EEG, MRI of the head, cardiovascular evaluation, and ECG were all normal. The following year he had a second brief (less than 1 minute) episode of loss of consciousness syncope while walking with his daughter on her college campus, again preceded by a brief moment of nausea. No tonic or clonic movements were observed, and there was no urinary incontinence. Following this episode, he underwent tilt-table testing with isoproterenol infusion. During testing, his heart rate dropped from 120 beats per minute to 80 beats per minute associated with nausea but without significant lightheadedness or syncope. He was treated with atenolol and fludrocortisone. Five months later, a third episode occurred while the patient was seated close to a camp fire. There was minimal warning and recovery was prompt. The dose of atenolol was increased. The fourth episode occurred 2 weeks before referral while the patient was driving. The patient suffered minor contusion on his forehead. Another driver reported that the patient was completely unresponsive when he first arrived at the scene, but the patient regained consciousness moments later.

Cardiovascular and neurologic examination, routine blood chemistry, ECG, 24-hour Holter with ambulatory blood pressure monitoring, response to carotid sinus massage, and EEG (both routine and sleep deprived) were normal. Tilt-table testing repeated without isoproterenol after discontinuation of fludrocortisone induced a typical vasovagal response after 38 minutes of head-up tilt associated with symptoms of blurred vision, diaphoresis, and presyncope that were not similar to his usual premonitory symptoms.

Because the symptoms induced during the vasovagal response were significantly different from the patient's spontaneous symptoms, the tilt-table test was not considered diagnostic. After detailed discussion, it was decided to proceed with an implantable loop recorder and discontinue use of atenolol. A form from the State Transportation Department was filed to recommend no driving. Three weeks after the loop recorder was implanted, another event occurred while the patient was seated at work. A coworker witnessed the event and activated the loop recorder (the patient had instructed all his coworkers on how to activate the loop recorder). The event recorder was interrogated and the stored electrogram is shown in Fig. 4. From a baseline regular sinus rhythm of approximately 60 bpm, there was a first pause that lasted for 2 seconds followed by two beats, an escape beat, then a pause of 13 seconds before normal rhythm returned. The diagnosis of intermittent sinus node dysfunction was documented. A dual chamber pacemaker was implanted. At the 3-month follow-up, the patient was

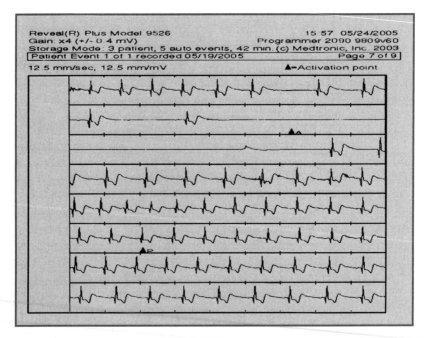

Fig. 4. A single lead electrogram was downloaded from the implantable loop recorder. The left column shows the actual time when the event was recorded. The paper speed is 12.5 mm/s. Each interval between two markers on the rhythm strip is 1 second.

doing well without any recurrence of syncope off all medications. A form to give permission to resume driving was forwarded to the transportation department.

This case emphasizes that the most important and fruitful elements of syncope evaluation are a detailed clinical history and a careful physical examination. The abrupt onset and immediate/complete recovery without any significant neurological sequelae are usually suggestive of a cardiogenic cause of syncope, but urinary incontinence is atypical and a thorough neurologic evaluation was therefore warranted. The results from the two tilt-table tests were judged to be falsely positive because the symptoms induced in the laboratory did not correlate with the patient's spontaneous symptoms. If symptoms induced during the tilt-table testing are significantly different from the clinical presentation, and a cardiac cause of syncope is considered likely, aggressive efforts must be made to establish a diagnosis.

Invasive electrophysiology evaluation versus implantable loop monitor

There are two principal approaches to the diagnosis of cardiac arrhythmias in patients with syncope. The first includes provocative studies, such as electrophysiologic testing, in an attempt to induce arrhythmias, which are responsible for clinical symptoms. The advantage of this approach is to provide the opportunity for immediate diagnostic conclusions and therapeutic recommendations according to the test results. The main disadvantage is the lack of evidence that the induced arrhythmia reflects the real clinical problem and the invasive nature of the approach. In this regard, the second approach of prolonged rhythm recording seems promising as a tool having the capability to display electrocardiographic tracings during an actual clinical event. The important limitation of this wait-and-watch strategy is the potential of subjecting patients to a certain degree of risk of trauma or even sudden death if the next episode is caused by malignant rhythm disturbances. Another obvious restriction of this approach is related to the limited value of Holter systems or any external electrocardiographic recorders or transmitters in the setting of usually infrequent, unpredictable, abrupt, and short-lived syncopal events.

Several questions should be addressed before subjecting a patient to invasive electrophysiology testing: (1) Is the information obtained from the history and noninvasive tests adequate to explain the patient's clinical presentation? (2) Could the results of invasive electrophysiology testing offer additional prognostic information? (3) Can the results of electrophysiology testing affect and guide therapy? The clinical judgment of an individual cardiac electrophysiologist is the critical determinant of the need for electrophysiology testing. The decision is primarily based on the relative probabilities of a cardiac cause of syncope and the projected diagnostic yield. In patients without underlying heart disease or any abnormalities on the ECG, the percentage in which an arrhythmogenic cause of unexplained syncope is disclosed by electrophysiology testing is generally low, ranging from 10% to 20% [2]. Although electrophysiology testing might have been indicated in this patient because of the recurrent and suspected cardiogenic nature of syncope, a positive diagnostic yield would have been low as this patient did not have any structural heart disease or any abnormalities on the ECG. Most instances of sinus node dysfunction due to a fixed substrate are invariably diagnosed by a noninvasive technique, such as ECG, Holter, or ambulatory loop recorder. The electrophysiology testing has limited diagnostic value in arrhythmogenic substrate of a transient nature.

The implantable loop recorder is capable of providing long-term (14–18 months) continuous rhythm monitoring and is particularly useful in patients with infrequent symptoms suspicious of an intermittent and transient arrhythmogenic substrate [25–27]. The device can be programmed to automatically record events outside of preset lower and upper heart rate limits or to patient-activated mode during an event. Subsequent interrogation provides a single lead electrogram with good quality. Several studies have reported the diagnostic efficacy of the implantable loop recorder in selected patient populations. The device is useful and most specific in documenting cardiac arrhythmias. It is less effective and specific in diagnosing vasovagal or hypotensive events as the device lacks the capability of providing blood pressure information [28].

Should this patient drive?

Although it has been estimated that approximately 40,000 deaths occur annually as a result of motor vehicle accidents in the United States, the exact frequency with which medical causes contribute to these accidents is not known. In Great Britain, it has been estimated that sudden driver incapacity has been reported with an incidence approximating 1/1,000 of all traffic accidents [29]. Most medical causes of road accidents occur in drivers who are already known to have preexisting diseases. Reports of 2,000 motor vehicle accidents involving loss of consciousness during driving (based on reports from the police to driver vehicle licensing agency in Great Britain) suggest that epilepsy is involved in 38% of cases, syncope in 21%, diabetes in 18%, heart condition in 8%, stroke in 7%, and other causes in 7%. The most recent recommendations for driving guidelines (European Society of Cardiology 2004) [2] in patients suffering from reflex syncope (vasovagal, carotid sinus hypersensitivity) suggest that patients with severe recurrent symptoms should not drive for 3 months once effective treatment has been initiated. Recommendations from AHA/NASPE on driving in patients with cardiac arrhythmias were last published in 1996 [30]. For the patient in the case example, driving was prohibited before the diagnosis because of the nature of the recurrent events. Following the diagnosis and treatment, the authors followed the suggestion that driving can be resumed after 3 months if syncope does not recur.

Case 5: recurrent syncope, weakness, and painful dysesthesia

A 38-year-old man presented with a 5-week history of painful dysesthesia and progressive weight loss of 15 kg. Routine clinical was normal, and the patient was referred to a rheumatologist for further evaluation. Because of the sensory symptoms, the patient was referred for nerve conductions and electromyography (EMG). A minimal sensorimotor axonal neuropathy was documented. The clinical examination performed in the EMG laboratory documented a history of increased dry mouth and hoarseness as well as erectile dysfunction with absence of early morning erections. The patient admitted to losing consciousness on two separate occasions within the previous 2 weeks. Physical examination documented presence of palmar and plantar hypohydrosis, miosis, resting tachycardia, and severe orthostatic hypotension.

Autonomic lab evaluation was performed that day. There was no sudomotor response to iontopheresed pilocarpine as measured by the silastic skin mold technique. There was no change in heart rate variability to rhythmic deep breathing. During the Valsalva maneuver there was a profound decrease in blood pressure during phase II of the maneuver with no evidence of overshoot during phase IV. The initial response to head-up tilt, as shown in Fig. 5, documented significant orthostatic hypotension with reduced compensatory tachycardia for the level of hypotension produced. A diagnosis of subacute autonomic neuropathy was made and the patient was treated with intravenous immunoglobulin (IvIg) 1 gm/kg/day on day 54 and 55 of his illness. The following tests were normal: biochemistry; CBC; antinuclear antibody (ANA), erythrocyte sedimentation rate (ESR), serum protein electrophoresis, serum immunoglobulins, urine Bence Jones protein, CD_3, CD_4, CD_8 count; thyroid stimulating hormone (TSH), T_4, cortisol, ACTH stimulation; Campylobacter, HIV and C. difficile cytotoxin, Lyme; blood protoporphyrins; CSF protein, glucose, IgG, oligoclonal bands, viral cultures; chest radiography, CT of the abdomen and pelvis; and bone scan.

Why was it difficult to make the diagnosis?

Although the case presentation depicts a seemingly obvious clinical presentation of subacute autonomic failure, the diagnosis of either subacute or progressive autonomic failure is often missed because early warning symptoms are not heeded and physical signs not appreciated. Syncope that is caused by orthostatic hypotension [31] or autonomic failure may be suggested by symptoms associated with standing alone or standing after meals or exercise. However, patients with chronic autonomic failure may not have symptoms of lightheadedness even with profound hypotension because cerebral autoregulation has adapted to compensate for large drops in blood pressure. In some instances the only symptom of profound orthostatic hypotension is a characteristic cervical pain or coat-hanger headache possibly

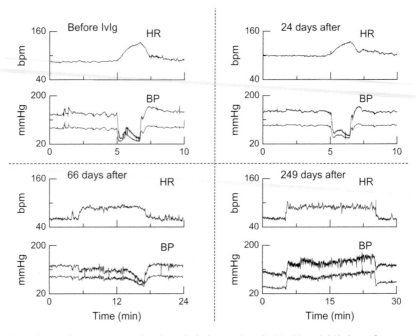

Fig. 5. Successive responses to head-up tilt before and again 11, 66, and 249 days after treatment with intravenous immunoglobulin. In each case, tilt occurs after 5 minutes of supine
rest. Note the progressive improvement in the response to head-up tilt with vasovagal syncope
after 10 minutes of tilt after 2 months, and a normal response after 9 months. HR, heart rate;
BP, blood pressure.

due to ischemia of the paracervical muscles. Other symptoms of autonomic
dysfunction, such as dry eyes or mouth, abnormal patterns of sweating, or
GI dysfunction, should be sought after. Blood pressure should be measured
after the patient has been supine for at least 5 minutes and then initially
upon standing and serially for at least 3 minutes. In some cases of early autonomic failure, orthostatic hypotension will only be detected when blood
pressure is measured in the upright position after food or exercise. Lack
of sweating of the palms or soles or significant truncal sweating in the absence of limb sweating (compensatory hyperhydrosis) at normal or cool ambient temperature may also suggest autonomic failure. Small-fiber sensory
neuropathy may be present if orthostatic hypotension is caused by postgan-
glionic autonomic neuropathy (as in this patient). Drugs that contribute to
orthostatic hypotension (most common cause of orthostatic hypotension)
must always be identified.

In this patient the subacute presentation of symptoms and evidence of
pandysautonomia on clinical and laboratory evaluation made the diagnosis
of subacute autonomic neuropathy likely. When making this diagnosis one
must carefully search for evidence of coexisting diseases or offending medications that may be associated with autonomic failure. A careful workup for

other autoimmune diseases or underlying malignancy associated with paraneoplastic autonomic neuropathy must also be performed. Diagnostic accuracy may often be improved by demonstrating high levels of serum neuronal
nicotininc acetylcholine antibodies [32].

Response to treatment

As shown in Fig. 5, no substantial change in autonomic evaluation was
noted on repeat evaluation day 11 following treatment. However, by day
24 of treatment, partial recovery of blood pressure was noted during late
phase II of the Valsalva maneuver, although orthostatic hypotension was
still present. By 4 months from the onset of illness (day 66 after treatment),
the profile of the Valsalva maneuver was nearly normal, and stand time had
increased to greater than 10 minutes. At this time the patient was able to exercise for 1 hour, to remain upright for prolonged periods, and to return to
full-time work the following month. Normal cardiovascular responses to
head-up tilt and the Valsalva maneuver were confirmed on two separate
evaluations done 147 and 249 days after treatment with IvIg.

Although there have been only a few case reports of positive response to
treatment of subacute autonomic neuropathy with IvIg, this mode of therapy should always be tried if the diagnosis can be made within a few months
of onset of the disease. Recovery from this condition is incomplete if left untreated. Even cases of apparently chronic autonomic failure may have an
autoimmune basis amenable to therapy [33].

Summary

In this series of clinical vignettes, the authors have attempted to provide
a "feel" for the varied causes of syncope. The neurologist should be able
to diagnose most causes of syncope using a simple algorithmic approach
[34, 35]. Initial evaluation includes detailed clinical history, physical examination, and 12-lead ECG. Following initial evaluation, the cause of syncope
is usually immediately apparent (typical story for vasovagal syncope, clinically demonstrable autonomic failure, long QT), strongly suspected (syncope
preceded by chest pain or palpitations), or uncertain. In the latter group of
patients, further workup will depend on the suspicion or documented presence of heart disease. In those with a single episode of syncope and no evidence of heart disease, further workup may not be necessary. In patients
over 60 years of age with recurrent episodes and no cardiac history or abnormal ECG, tilt-table testing and carotid sinus massage may be diagnostic. If
no diagnosis is found, an implantable loop monitor may be needed. Patients
with heart disease will need the most comprehensive evaluations, possibly including exercise testing, cardiac electrophysiology, and tilt-table testing. As
better understanding of pathophysiology and epidemiology emerge, understanding of the diagnosis and treatment of syncope will improve. In the
meantime, there is no substitute for astute clinical acumen.

References

[1] van Dijk JG. Explaining syncope: faints need not confuse. Europace 2005;7(4):392–5.

[2] Brignole M, Alboni P, Benditt DG, Bergfeldt L, Blanc JJ, Bloch Thomsen PE, et al. Guidelines on management (diagnosis and treatment) of syncope—update 2004. Europace 2004; 6(6):467–537.

[3] Graham LA, Kenny RA. Clinical characteristics of patients with vasovagal reactions presenting as unexplained syncope. Europace 2001;3(2):141–6.

[4] Mathias CJ, Deguchi K, Bleasdale-Barr K, Kimber JR. Frequency of family history in vasovagal syncope. Lancet 1998;352(9121):33–4.

[5] Mathias CJ, Deguchi K, Schatz I. Observations on recurrent syncope and presyncope in 641 patients. Lancet 2001;357(9253):348–53.

[6] Alboni P, Brignole M, Menozzi C, Raviele A, Del Rosso A, Dinelli M, et al. Diagnostic value of history in patients with syncope with or without heart disease. J Am Coll Cardiol 2001; 37(7):1921–8.

[7] Oh JH, Hanusa BH, Kapoor WN. Do symptoms predict cardiac arrhythmias and mortality in patients with syncope? Arch Intern Med 1999;159(4):375–80.

[8] Kapoor WN, Hanusa BH. Is syncope a risk factor for poor outcomes? Comparison of patients with and without syncope. Am J Med 1996;100(6):646–55.

[9] Sheldon R, Rose S, Connolly S, Ritchie D, Koshman ML, Frenneaux M. Diagnostic criteria for vasovagal syncope based on a quantitative history. Eur Heart J 2006;27(3):344–50.

[10] Sheldon R, Rose S, Ritchie D, Connolly SJ, Koshman M-L, Lee MA, et al. Historical criteria that distinguish syncope from seizures. J Am Coll Cardiol 2002;40(1):142–8.

[11] van Lieshout JJ, Wieling W, Karemaker JM, Eckberg DL. The vasovagal response. Clin Sci 1991;81(5):575–86.

[12] Kapoor WN, Brant N. Evaluation of syncope by upright tilt testing with isoproterenol. A nonspecific test. Ann Intern Med 1992;116(5):358–63.

[13] Benditt DG, Ferguson DW, Grubb BP, Kapoor WN, Kugler J, Lerman BB, et al. Tilt table testing for assessing syncope. J Am Coll Cardiol 1996;28(1):263–75.

[14] Krediet CTP, van Dijk N, Linzer M, van Lieshout JJ, Wieling W. Management of vasovagal syncope: controlling or aborting faints by leg crossing and muscle tensing. Circulation 2002; 106(13):1684–9.

[15] The Task Force on Syncope ESoC. Guidelines on management (diagnosis and treatment) of syncope— update 2004. Europace 2004;6(6):467–537.

[16] Sheldon R, Rose S, Connolly S. Prevention of Syncope Trial (POST): a randomized clinical trial of beta blockers in the prevention of vasovagal syncope: rationale and study design. Europace 2003;5(1):71–5.

[17] Raviele A, Brignole M, Sutton R, Alboni P, Giani P, Menozzi C, et al. Effect of etilefrine in preventing syncopal recurrence in patients with vasovagal syncope: a double-blind, randomized, placebo-controlled trial. The Vasovagal Syncope International Study. Circulation 1999;99(11):1452–7.

[18] Connolly SJ, Sheldon R, Roberts RS, Gent M. Vasovagal Pacemaker Study I. The North American Vasovagal Pacemaker Study (VPS)—A randomized trial of permanent cardiac pacing for the prevention of vasovagal syncope. J Am Coll Cardiol 1999;33(1): 16–20.

[19] Connolly SJ, Sheldon R, Thorpe KE, Roberts RS, Ellenbogen KA, Wilkoff BL, et al. Pacemaker therapy for prevention of syncope in patients with recurrent severe vasovagal syncope. Second Vasovagal Pacemaker Study (VPS II): a randomized trial. JAMA 2003; 289(17):2224–9.

[20] Kaufmann H, Saadia D, Voustianiouk A. Midodrine in neurally mediated syncope: a double-blind, crossover study. Ann Neurol 2002;52(3):342–5.

[21] Di Girolamo E, Di Iorio C, Sabatini P, Leonzio L, Barbone C, Barsotti A. Effects of paroxetine hydrochloride, a selective serotonin reuptake inhibitor on refractory vasovagal

syncope: a randomized, double-blind, placebo controlled study. J Am Coll Cardiol 1999; 33(5):1227–30.

[22] Chen LY, Gersh BJ, Hodge DO, Wieling W, Hammill SC, Shen WK. Prevalence and clinical outcomes of patients with multiple potential causes of syncope. Mayo Clin Proc 2003;78(4): 414–20.

[23] Brady PA, Shen WK. When is intracardiac electrophysiologic evaluation indicated in the older or very elderly patient? Complications rates and data. Clin Geriatr Med 2002;18(2): 339–60.

[24] Shen WK, Decker WW, Smars PA, Goyal DG, Walker AE, Hodge DO, Trusty JM, et al. Syncope Evaluation in the Emergency Department Study (SEEDS): a multidisciplinary approach to syncope management. Circulation 2004;110(23):3636–45.

[25] Krahn AD, Klein GJ, Yee R, Manda V. The high cost of syncope: cost implications of a new insertable loop recorder in the investigation of recurrent syncope. Am Heart J 1999;137(5): 870–7.

[26] Krahn AD, Klein GJ, Skanes AC, Yee R. Insertable loop recorder use for detection of intermittent arrhythmias. Pacing Clin Electrophysiol 2004;27(5):657–64.

[27] Armstrong VL, Lawson J, Kamper AM, Newton J, Kenny RA. The use of an implantable loop recorder in the investigation of unexplained syncope in the older people. Age Ageing 2003;82(2):185–8.

[28] Luria DM, Shen WK. Syncope in the elderly: New trends in diagnostic approach and nonpharmacologic management. Am J Geriatr Cardiol 2001;10(2):91–6.

[29] Petch MC. Driving and heart disease. Eur Heart J 1998;19(8):1165–77.

[30] Epstein AE, Miles WN, Benditt DG, Camm JA, Darling EJ, Friedman PL, et al. Personal and public safety issues related to arrhythmias that may affect consciousness: applications for regulation and physician advice. Circulation 1996;94(5):1147–66.

[31] The Consensus Committee of the American Autonomic Society and the American Academy of Neurology. The definition of orthostatic hypotension, pure autonomic failure and multiple system atrophy. Neurology 1996;46(5):1470.

[32] Vernino S, Adamski J, Kryzer TJ, Fealey RD, Lennon VA. Neuronal nicotinic ACh receptor antibody in subacute autonomic neuropathy and cancer-related syndromes. Neurology 1998;50(6):1806–13.

[33] Schroeder C, Vernino S, Birkenfeld AL, Tank J, Heusser K, Lipp A, et al. Plasma exchange for primary autoimmune autonomic failure. N Engl J Med 2005;353(15):1585–90.

[34] Kaufmann H, Wieling W. Syncope: a clinically guided diagnostic algorithm. Clin Auton Res 2004;14(Suppl):187–90.

[35] Brignole M, Menozzi C, Bartoletti A, Giada F, Lagi A, Ungar A, et al. A new management of syncope: prospective systematic guideline-based evaluation of patients referred urgently to general hospitals. Eur Heart J 2006;27(1):76–82.

NEUROLOGIC
CLINICS

Neurol Clin 24 (2006) 233–265

ELSEVIER
SAUNDERS

Neuromuscular Disorders in Clinical Practice: Case Studies

Jay R. Bhatt, MD, Robert M. Pascuzzi, MD*

*Department of Neurology, Indiana University School of Medicine,
1120 South Drive, Indianapolis, IN 46202, USA*

Neuromuscular disorders represent a large group of highly varied and interesting clinical disorders, many of which have major general medical manifestations. These disorders can be diagnosed largely based on the patient's history and physical examination with a little help from modern technology. Despite the outdated belief that neurologic conditions are diagnosed but rarely treatable, all cases discussed herein represent disorders for which there are extensive options and opportunities for meaningful management. These 16 brief case overviews challenge and refresh diagnostic skills and provide the framework for selected comments regarding management options.

Case 1: Myasthenia Gravis

This 27-year-old woman presented with 3 months of episodic fluctuating double vision and droopy eyelids (Fig. 1). When she is tired or in the heat or humidity, her symptoms become worse. In general she is better earlier in the day. The week of presentation she developed slurred speech and difficulty swallowing. The exam shows facial appearance as in Fig. 1. Neck flexion and extension are mildly weak, as are the proximal limb muscles. Sensation and reflexes are normal. What is the diagnosis, how is it confirmed, and how should she be managed?

Discussion

Myasthenia gravis (MG) is an autoimmune disorder of neuromuscular transmission involving the production of autoantibodies directed against the nicotinic acetylcholine receptor [1–3]. Acetylcholine receptor antibodies

---

* Corresponding author.
E-mail address: prcowher@iupui.edu (R.M. Pascuzzi).

0733-8619/06/$ - see front matter © 2006 Elsevier Inc. All rights reserved.
doi:10.1016/j.ncl.2006.01.011   *neurologic.theclinics.com*

Fig. 1. Edrophonium chloride test: baseline; 30 s after 3 mg edrophonium IV, looking up 1 min later, looking up 3 min later (dysconjugate gaze), and 5 min after infusion (severe ptosis, bifacial weakness, and dysconjugate gaze).

are detectable in the serum of 80% to 90% of patients with MG. The prevalence of MG is about 1 in 10,000 to 20,000. Women are affected about twice as often as men. Symptoms may begin at virtually any age with a peak in women in the second and third decades; the peak in men occurs in the fifth and sixth decades. Associated autoimmune diseases, such as rheumatoid arthritis, lupus, and pernicious anemia, are present in about 5% of patients. Thyroid disease occurs in about 10%, often in association with antithyroid antibodies. About 10% to 15% of MG patients have a thymoma, and thymic lymphoid hyperplasia with proliferation of germinal centers occurs in 50% to 70% of cases.

Clinical Features

The hallmark of MG is fluctuating or fatigable weakness. The presenting symptoms are ocular in half of all patients (25% of patients initially present with diplopia, 25% with ptosis) and by one month into the course of illness, 80% of patients have some degree of ocular involvement. Presenting symptoms are bulbar (dysarthria or dysphagia) in 10%, leg weakness (impaired walking) in 10%, and generalized weakness in 10%. Respiratory failure is the presenting symptom in 1% of cases. Patients usually complain of symptoms from focal muscle dysfunction, such as diplopia, ptosis, dysarthria, dysphagia, to inability to work with arms raised over the head to disturbance of gait. Patients with MG tend not to complain of generalized weakness, generalized fatigue, sleepiness, or muscle pain. In the classic case, fluctuating weakness is worse with exercise and improved with rest. Symptoms tend to progress later in the day. Many different factors can precipitate or aggravate weakness, such as physical stress, emotional stress, infection, or exposure to medications that impair neuromuscular transmission (perioperative succinylcholine, aminoglycoside antibiotics, quinine, qunidine, botulinum toxin).

Diagnosis

The diagnosis is based on a history of fluctuating weakness with corroborating findings on examination. There are several ways to validate or confirm the clinical diagnosis. Improvement following administration of cholinesterase inhibitors, such as edrophonium, has an estimated sensitivity of 80% to 90% with good but not perfect specificity (improvement following IV edrophonium has been reported in other neuromuscular diseases, including Lambert Eaton syndrome, botulism, Guillain-Barré syndrome, motor neuron disease, and lesions of the brainstem and cavernous sinus). Acetylcholine receptor-binding antibodies are present in about 80% of all myasthenia patients (50% of patients with pure ocular MG, 80% of those with mild generalized MG, 90% of patients with moderate to severe generalized MG, and 70% of those in clinical remission). By also testing for modulating and blocking antibodies, the sensitivity improves to 90% overall. Specificity is outstanding, with false positives exceedingly rare in reliable labs.

More recently, about a third of MG patients seronegative for acetylcholine receptor antibodies have been shown to have muscle-specific kinase (MuSK) antibodies. MuSK antibodies can now be measured by a commercially available immunoprecipitation assay. The clinical features of MuSK-positive patients may differ from non-MuSK MG patients. Such patients tend to be younger women (under age 40) with lower likelihood of abnormal repetitive stimulation and edrophonium test results. Bulbar symptoms are significantly more common at onset of disease in MuSK antibody positive patients. MuSK antibodies may also be more commonly associated with patients having weakness of neck extensor, shoulders, or respiratory muscles.

Repetitive stimulation testing is widely available and has variable sensitivity, depending on number and selection of muscles studied and various provocative maneuvers. However, in most labs this technique has a sensitivity of about 50% in all patients with MG (lower in patients with mild or pure ocular disease). In general, the yield from repetitive stimulation is higher when testing muscle groups having clinically significant weakness. Single-fiber electromyography (SFEMG) is a highly specialized technique, usually available in major academic centers, with a sensitivity of about 90%. Abnormal single-fiber results are common in other neuromuscular diseases and therefore the test must be used in the correct clinical context. The specificity of single-fiber EMG is an important issue in that mild abnormalities can clearly be present with various other diseases of the motor unit, including motor neuron disease, peripheral neuropathy, and myopathy. Disorders of neuromuscular transmission other than MG can have substantial abnormalities on SFEMG. In contrast, acetylcholine receptor antibodies (and MuSK antibodies) are not found in non-MG patients. In summary, the two highly sensitive laboratory studies are single-fiber EMG and acetylcholine receptor antibodies; however, neither test is 100% sensitive.

Treatment

Appropriate management of the patient with autoimmune MG requires understanding of the natural course of the disease (Box 1 and 2). The long-term natural course of MG is not clearly established other than being highly variable. Several generalizations can be made. About half of MG patients present with ocular symptoms and by 1 month 80% have eye findings. The presenting weakness is bulbar in 10%, limb in 10%, generalized in

Box 1. General guidelines for management

1. Be certain of the diagnosis.
2. Provide patient education. Inform the patient about the natural course of the disease (including the variable and somewhat unpredictable course). Briefly review the treatment options outlined above pointing out effectiveness, time course of improvement, duration of response, and complications. Provide the patient with educational pamphlets prepared by the Myasthenia Gravis Foundation of America or the Muscular Dystrophy Association.
3. Know when to hospitalize the patient. Patients with severe MG can deteriorate rapidly over a period of hours. Therefore, those having dyspnea should be hospitalized immediately in a constant observation or intensive care setting. Patients with moderate or severe dysphagia, weight loss, and those with rapidly progressive or severe weakness should be admitted urgently. This will allow close monitoring and early intervention in the case of respiratory failure, and will also expedite the diagnostic workup and initiation of therapy.
4. Myasthenic crisis is a medical emergency characterized by respiratory failure from diaphragm weakness or severe oropharyngeal weakness leading to aspiration. Crisis can occur in the setting of surgery (postop), acute infection, or following rapid withdrawal of corticosteroids (though some patients have no precipitating factors). Patients should be placed in an ICU setting and have forced vital capacity (FVC) checked every 2 hours. Changes in arterial blood gases occur late in neuromuscular respiratory failure. There should a low threshold for intubation and mechanical ventilation. Criteria for intubation include a drop in the FVC below 15 ml/kg (or below 1 liter in an average-sized adult), severe aspiration from oropharyngeal weakness, or labored breathing regardless of the measurements. If the diagnosis is not clear-cut it is advisable to secure the airway with intubation, stabilize ventilation, and only then address the question of the underlying diagnosis. If the patient has been taking a cholinesterase inhibitor (CEI), the drug should be temporarily discontinued to rule out the possibility of cholinergic crisis.
5. Screen for and correct any underlying medical problems, such as systemic infection, metabolic problems (like diabetes), and thyroid disease (hypo- or hyperthyroidism can exacerbate MG).

6. Know which drugs to avoid in MG. Avoid using
d-penicillamine, alfa-interferon, chloroquine, quinine,
quinidine, procainamide, and botulinum toxin.
Aminoglycoside antibiotics should be avoided unless needed
for a life-threatening infection. Neuromuscular blocking drugs,
such as pancuronium and D-tubocurarine, can produce
marked and prolonged paralysis in MG patients. Depolarizing
drugs, such as succinylcholine, can also have a prolonged
effect and should be used by a skilled anesthesiologist who is
aware of the patient's MG.

10%, and respiratory in 1%. By 1 month, symptoms remain purely ocular in 40%, generalized in 40%, limited to the limbs in 10%, and limited to bulbar muscles in 10%. Weakness remains restricted to the ocular muscles on a long-term basis in about 15% to 20% (pure ocular MG). Most patients with initial ocular involvement tend to develop generalized weakness within the first year of the disease (90% of those who generalize do so within the initial 12 months). Maximal weakness occurs within the initial 3 years in 70% of patients. Death from MG is rare. Spontaneous long-lasting remission occurs in about 10 to 15%, usually in the first year or two of the disease. Most MG patients develop progression of clinical symptoms during the initial 2 to 3 years. However, progression is not uniform, as illustrated by 15% to 20% of patients whose symptoms remain purely ocular and those who have spontaneous remission.

Cholinesterase Inhibitors

Cholinesterase inhibitors (CEI) are safe, effective, and first-line therapy in all patients. Inhibition of acetylcholinesterase (AChE) reduces the hydrolysis of acetylcholine (ACh), increasing the accumulation of ACh at the nicotinic postsynaptic membrane. The CEIs used in MG bind reversibly (as opposed to organophosphate CEIs, which bind irreversibly) to AChE. These drugs cross the blood-brain barrier poorly and tend not to cause central nervous system side effects. Absorption from the gastrointestinal tract tends to be inefficient and variable, with oral bioavailability of about 10%. Muscarinic autonomic side effects, including gastrointestinal cramping, diarrhea, salivation, lacrimation, diaphoresis, and, when severe, bradycardia, may occur with all of the CEI preparations. A feared potential complication of excessive CEI use is skeletal muscle weakness (cholinergic weakness). Patients receiving parenteral CEI are at the greatest risk to have cholinergic weakness. It is uncommon for patients receiving oral CEI to develop significant cholinergic weakness even while experiencing muscarinic cholinergic side effects. Commonly available CEIs are summarized in Table 1.

Box 2. Myasthenia gravis: Guidelines for specific therapies

Treatment must be individualized. Mild diplopia and ptosis may not be disabling for some patients, but for a pilot or neurosurgeon, mild intermittent diplopia may be critical. In similar fashion, some patients may tolerate side effects better than others.

- Mild or trivial weakness, localized or generalized, should be managed with a cholinesterase inhibitor (CEI) (pyridostigmine).
- Moderate to marked weakness, localized or generalized, should initially be managed with CEIs. Even if symptoms are adequately controlled, patients under age 55 undergo thymectomy early in the course of the disease (within the first year). In older patients thymectomy is usually not performed unless the patient is thought to have a thymoma. Thymectomy is performed at an experienced center with the clear intent of complete removal of the gland. All patients with suspected thymoma (by chest scan) should have thymectomy, even if their myasthenic symptoms are mild. Unless a thymoma is suspected, patients with pure ocular disease are usually not treated with thymectomy.
- If symptoms are inadequately controlled on CEIs, immunosuppression is used. High-dose corticosteroid therapy is the most predictable and effective long-term option. If patients have severe, rapidly progressive, or life-threatening symptoms the decision to start corticosteroids is clear cut. Patients with disabling but stable symptoms may instead receive mycophenolate mofetil especially if there are particular concerns about using corticosteroids (ie, the patient is already overweight, diabetic, or cosmetic concerns). Those patients who respond poorly or have unacceptable complications on steroids are started on mycophenolate.
- Plasma exchange or IVIG are indicated in
  - rapidly progressive, life-threatening, impending myasthenic crisis or actual crisis, particularly if prolonged intubation with mechanical ventilation is judged hazardous;
  - preoperative stabilization of MG (such as prior to thymectomy or other elective surgery) in poorly controlled patients; and
  - disabling MG refractory to other therapies.
- If these options fail, then azathioprine or cyclosporine is recommended.
- If the patient remains poorly controlled despite treatment as above, then perform a repeat chest CT scan looking for

residual thymus. Some patients improve after repeat thymectomy. Check for other medical problems (diabetes, thyroid disease, infection, and coexisting autoimmune diseases).

- Referral to a neurologist or center specializing in neuromuscular disease is advised for all patients with suspected MG and can be particularly important for complicated or refractory patients.

Pyridostigmine

Pyridostigmine is the most widely used CEI for long-term oral therapy. Onset of effect is within 15 to 30 minutes of an oral dose, with peak effect within 1 to 2 hours. Wearing off begins gradually at 3 to 4 hours postdose. The starting dose is 30 to 60 mg three to four times per day, depending on symptoms. Optimal benefit usually occurs with a dose of 60 mg every 4 hours. Muscarinic cholinergic side effects are common with larger doses. Occasional patients require and tolerate over 1,000 mg/day, dosing as frequently as every 2 to 3 hours. Patients with significant bulbar weakness will often time their dose about 1 hour before meals to maximize chewing and swallowing. Of all the CEI preparations pyridostigmine has the least

Table 1
Cholinesterase inhibitors

	Unit dose	Average dose
Adult dosing:		
Pyridostigmine bromide tablet	60 mg tablet	30–60 mg every 4–6 h
Pyridostigmine bromide syrup	12 mg/ml	30–60 mg every 4–6 h
Pyridostigmine bromide extended release	180-mg tablet	1 tablet twice daily
Pyridostigmine bromide (parenteral)	5-mg/ml ampoules	1–2 mg every 3–4 h (1/30 of oral dose)
Neostigmine bromide	15-mg tablet	7.5–15 mg every 3–4 h
Neostigmine methylsulfate (parenteral)	0.25–1.0-mg/ml ampoules	0.5 mg IM, IV, or SC every 2–3 h
Children's dosing:		
Edrophonium		
Diagnosis: 0.1 mg/Kg IV (or 0.15 mg/Kg IM or SC, which prolongs the effect), preceded by a test dose of 0.01 mg/Kg		
Pyridostigmine bromide		
Treatment: Oral dose is about 1.0 mg/Kg every 4–6 hours, as tablets or syrup (60 mg/5 ml)		
Neostigmine methylsulfate (parenteral)		
Diagnosis: 0.1 mg/Kg/ IM or SC X1 or 0.05 mg/Kg/ IV X1		
Treatment: 0.01–0.04 mg/Kg/dose IM, IV, or SC q 2–3 as needed		

Abbreviations: IM, intramuscular; IV, intravenous; SC, subcutaneous.

muscarinic side effects. Pyridostigmine may be used in several alternative forms to the 60-mg tablet. The syrup may be necessary for children or for patients who have difficulty swallowing pills. Sustained-release pyridostigmine 180 mg is sometimes preferred for nighttime use. Unpredictable release and absorption limit its use. Patients with severe dysphagia or those undergoing surgical procedures may need parenteral CEI. Intravenous pyridostigmine should be given at about 1/30 of the oral dose. Neostigmine (prostigmine) has a slightly shorter duration of action and slightly greater muscarinic side effects.

For patients with intolerable muscarinic side effects at CEI doses required for optimal power, a concomitant anticholinergic drug such as atropine sulfate (0.4–0.5 mg orally) or glycopyrrolate (1–2 mg orally) on a needed basis or with each dose of CEI may be helpful. Patients with mild disease can often be managed adequately with CEIs. However, patients with moderate, severe, or progressive disease usually require more effective therapy.

Thymectomy

Association of the thymus gland with MG was first noted around 1900, and thymectomy has become standard therapy for over 50 years. Prospective controlled trials have not been performed for thymectomy (although such a trial is currently in the planning stage). Nonetheless, thymectomy is generally recommended for patients with moderate to severe MG, especially those inadequately controlled on CEI and those under age 55 years. All patients with suspected thymoma undergo surgery. About 75% of MG patients appear to benefit from thymectomy. Patients may improve or simply stabilize. For unclear reasons the onset of improvement tends to be delayed by a year or two in most patients (some patients seem to improve 5 to 10 years after surgery). Most centers use the transsternal approach for thymectomy with the goal of complete removal including "maximal thymectomy" to ensure complete removal. If thymectomy is to be performed, choose an experienced surgeon, anesthesiologist, and center with a good track record and insist that the entire gland is removed.

Corticosteroids

There are no controlled trials documenting the benefit of corticosteroids in MG. However, nearly all authorities have personal experience attesting to the virtues (and complications) of corticosteroid use in MG patients. In general, corticosteroids are used in patients with moderate to severe disabling symptoms that are refractory to CEI. Patients are commonly hospitalized to initiate therapy because of the risk of early exacerbation. Opinions differ regarding the best method of administration. For patients with severe MG it is best to begin with high-dose daily oral therapy of 60 to 80 mg. Early exacerbation occurs in about half of patients, usually within the first few days of therapy and typically lasting 3 or 4 days. In 10% of cases the exacerbation is severe, requiring mechanical ventilation or a feeding tube (thus the need to initiate therapy in the hospital). Overall, about 80% of patients show a favorable response to steroids (with 30% attaining remission and 50% marked improvement). Mild to moderate improvement occurs in 15%, and 5% have no response. Improvement begins as early as 12 hours and as late as 60 days after beginning prednisone, but usually the patient begins to improve within the first week or two. Improvement is gradual, with marked improvement occurring at a mean of 3 months, and maximal improvement at a mean of 9 months. Of those patients having a favorable response, most maintain their improvement with gradual dosage reduction at a rate of 10 mg every 1 to 2 months. More rapid reduction is usually associated with a flair-up of the disease. Though many patients can eventually be weaned off of steroids and maintain their response, most cannot. They require a minimum dose (5–30 mg on alternate days) to maintain their improvement. Complications of long-term high-dose prednisone therapy are substantial and include Cushingoid appearance, hypertension, osteoporosis, cataracts, aseptic necrosis, and the other well-known complications of chronic steroid therapy. Older patients tend to respond more favorably to prednisone.

Alternative Immunosuppressive Drug Therapy

Mycophenolate Mofetil

Mycophenolate mofetil is a purine inhibitor widely used in recent years for the treatment of MG. Though prospective controlled trials are underway, anecdotal uncontrolled experience would suggest that about 75% of MG patients benefit from the drug with the typical onset of improvement within 2 to 3 months. The drug is in general well tolerated. Typically dosages begin at 250 to 500 mg twice a day orally, increasing over 2 to 4 weeks to 1,000 mg twice a day.

Azathioprine

Azathioprine is a cytotoxic purine analog with extensive use in MG (but largely uncontrolled and retrospective). The starting dose is 50 mg/day, with complete blood count and liver function tests weekly in the beginning. If the drug is tolerated and the blood work is stable, the dose is increased by 50 mg every 1 to 2 weeks, aiming for a total daily dose of 2 to 3 mg/kg/day (about 150 mg/day in the average-size adult). When azathioprine is first started, about 15% of patients will have intolerable gastrointestinal side effects (nausea, anorexia, abdominal discomfort), sometimes associated with fever, leading to discontinuation. Bone marrow suppression with relative leukopenia (white blood cell count [WBC] 2,500–4,000) occurs in 25% of patients but is usually not significant. If the WBC drops below 2,500 or the absolute granulocyte count goes below 1,000, the drug is stopped (and the abnormalities usually resolve). Macrocytosis is common and of unclear clinical significance. Liver enzymes elevate in 5% to 10% of patients, but this condition is usually reversible, and severe hepatic toxicity occurs in only about 1% of patients. Infection occurs in about 5%. There is a theoretical risk of malignancy (based on observations in organ transplant patients), but this increased risk has not been clearly established in the MG patient population. About half of MG patients improve on azathioprine, with onset 4 to 8 months into treatment. Maximal improvement takes about 12 months. Relapse after discontinuation of azathioprine occurs in over half of patients, usually within 1 year.

Cyclosporine

Cyclosporine is used in patients with severe MG who cannot adequately be managed with corticosteroids or azathioprine. The starting dose is 3 to 5 mg/kg/day given in two divided doses. Cyclosporine blood levels should be measured monthly (aiming for a level of 200–300) along with electrolytes, magnesium, and renal function (in general, serum creatinine should not exceed 1.5 times the pretreatment level). Blood should be sampled before the morning dose is taken. Over half of patients improve on cyclosporine. The onset of clinical improvement occurs about 1 to 2 months after beginning therapy, and maximal improvement occurs at about 3 to 4 months. Side effects include renal toxicity and hypertension. Nonsteroidal anti-inflammatory drugs and potassium-sparing diuretics are among the list of drugs that should be avoided while on cyclosporine. In patients on corticosteroids, the addition of cyclosporine can lead to a reduction in steroid dosage (although it is usually not possible to discontinue prednisone).

Plasma Exchange

Plasma exchange (plasmapheresis) removes acetylcholine receptor antibodies and results in rapid clinical improvement. The standard course involves removal of 2 to 3 L of plasma every other day or three times per week until the patient improves (usually a total of three to five exchanges). Improvement begins after the first few exchanges and reaches maximum within 2 to 3 weeks. The improvement is moderate to marked in nearly all patients but usually wears off after 4 to 8 weeks as a result of the reaccumulation of pathogenic antibodies. Vascular access may require placement of a central line. Complications include hypotension, bradycardia, electrolyte imbalance, hemolysis, infection, and access problems (such as pneumothorax from placement of a central line.) Indications for plasma exchange include any patient in whom a rapid temporary clinical improvement is needed.

High-Dose IVIG

High-dose intravenous immunoglobulin (IVIG) administration is associated with rapid improvement in MG symptoms in a time frame similar to plasma exchange. The mechanism is unclear but may relate to downregulation of acetylcholine receptor antibody production or to the effect of anti-idiotype antibodies. The usual protocol is 2 g/kg spread out over 5 consecutive days (0.4 g/kg/day). Different IVIG preparations are administered at different rates (contact the pharmacy for guidelines). Most MG patients improve, usually within 1 week of starting IVIG.

Case 2: Lambert Eaton Syndrome

This 35-year-old woman presented with 6 months of trouble walking, going up and down stairs, and rising from a sitting position (Fig. 2). She also experiences difficulty lifting items over her head and tires while washing her hair. She describes a dry mouth and a metallic taste. Exam shows 4/5 proximal weakness more pronounced in the lower extremities. She also has mild bifacial weakness and slight ptosis. Sensation is normal. Muscle stretch reflexes are absent. Lab studies show normal muscle enzymes. What is the diagnosis, how is it confirmed, and what is the best management of this patient?

Discussion

Lambert Eaton syndrome (LES) (myasthenic syndrome) is a presynaptic disease characterized by chronic fluctuating weakness of proximal limb muscles [4,5]. Symptoms include difficulty walking, climbing stairs, or rising from a chair (Box 3). In LES there may be some improvement in power with sustained or repeated exercise. In contrast, the myasthenia gravis ptosis, diplopia, dysphagia and respiratory failure are far less common. LES patients often complain of myalgias, muscle stiffness of the back and legs, distal paresthesias, metallic taste, dry mouth, impotence, and other autonomic symptoms of muscarinic cholinergic insufficiency. LES is rare

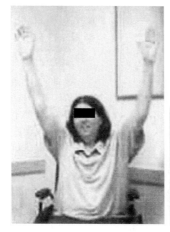
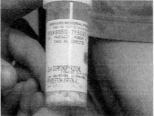

Fig. 2. Patient can lift up her arms after treatment with 3,4-diaminopyridine.

Box 3. Lambert Eaton syndrome

Symptoms
Proximal limb weakness
   Legs more commonly affected than arms
Fatigue or fluctuating symptoms
Difficulty rising from a sitting position, climbing stairs
Metallic taste in mouth
Autonomic dysfunction
   Dry mouth
   Constipation
   Blurred vision
   Impaired sweating

Signs
Proximal limb weakness
   Legs more commonly affected than arms
Weakness on exam is less pronounced compared with patient's
   level of disability
Hypoactive or absent muscle stretch reflexes
Lambert's sign (grip becomes more powerful over several
   seconds)

---

compared with myasthenia gravis, which is about 100 times more common. About half of LES patients have an underlying malignancy—usually small cell carcinoma of the lung. In patients without malignancy, LES is an autoimmune disease and can be associated with other autoimmune phenomenon. In general, patients over age 40 are more likely to be men and have an associated malignancy, whereas younger patients are more likely to be women and have no neoplasm malignancy. LES symptoms can precede detection of the malignancy by 1 to 2 years.

The examination typically shows proximal lower extremity weakness (although the objective bedside assessment may suggest mild weakness relative to the patient's history). The muscle stretch reflexes are absent. On testing sustained maximal grip there is a gradual increase in power over the initial 2 to 3 seconds (Lambert's sign).

The diagnosis is confirmed with EMG studies, which typically show low amplitude of the compound muscle action potentials and a decrement to slow rates or repetitive stimulation. Following brief exercise, there is marked facilitation of the CMAP amplitude. At high rates of repetitive stimulation, there may be an incremental response. Single-fiber EMG is markedly abnormal in virtually all patients with LES. The pathogenesis involves autoantibodies directed against voltage-gated calcium channels at cholinergic nerve terminals. These IgG antibodies also inhibit cholinergic synapses of the autonomic nervous system. Over 75% of LES patients demonstrated these antibodies to voltage-gated calcium channels in serum, providing another useful diagnostic test.

In patients with associated malignancy, successful treatment of the tumor can lead to improvement in the LES symptoms if the malignancy is successfully treated. Symptomatic improvement in neuromuscular transmission may occur with the use of cholinesterase inhibitors such as pyridostigmine. Guanidine has shown some benefit, but its use has been limited by bone marrow, renal, and hepatic toxicity. Guanidine increases the release of ACh by increasing the duration of the action potential at the motor nerve terminal. 3,4-diaminopyridine (DAP) increases ACh release by blocking voltage-dependent potassium conductance and thereby prolonging depolarization at the nerve terminal and enhancing the voltage-dependent calcium influx. 3,4 DAP has been shown to clearly improve most patients with LES with mild toxicity and is becoming increasingly available, such that it represents first-line symptomatic therapy for LES. The typical beginning dose is 10 mg every 4 to 6 hours with gradual increase as needed up to a maximum of 100 mg/day.

Immunosuppressive therapy is used in patients with disabling symptoms. Long-term high-dose corticosteroids, plasma exchange, and IVIG have all been used with moderate success. In general, the use of these therapies should be tailored to the severity of patient's symptoms.

The patient presented in this case has no associated malignancy. She has typical EMG findings and calcium channel antibodies and is managed successfully with long-term 3,4 DAP.

Case 3: Amyotrophic Lateral Sclerosis

This 45-year-old man presented with 12 months of gradual progressive painless loss of function and atrophy of the right arm and hand (Fig. 3). Over the past 6 months he has experienced similar weakness and atrophy creeping into the left arm and hand as well as the development of slurred speech and trouble swallowing liquids. Exam shows severe weakness and atrophy in the arms and tongue, fasciculations, and hyperactive muscle stretch reflexes. Sensation is normal. What is your diagnosis?

Discussion

Amyotrophic lateral sclerosis (ALS) is a slowly progressive disorder that affects motor neurons that are located in the brain and spinal cord [6]. The disease produces variable patterns of gradual progressive weakness in the muscles of the limbs, trunk, and those affecting speech, swallowing, and breathing. Amyotrophic lateral sclerosis, Lou Gehrig's disease, and motor neuron disease are all terms used interchangeably in common clinical practice.

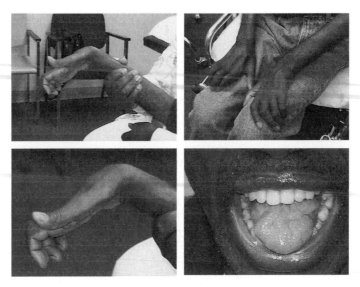

Fig. 3. Amyotrophic lateral sclerosis patient.

By definition, amyotrophic lateral sclerosis involves a gradual progressive malfunction of the upper motor neurons and also the lower motor neurons. Technically, if a patient has just involvement of the lower motor neurons, the disorder is called anterior horn cell disease or spinomuscular atrophy. Pure upper motor neuron disease is referred to as primary lateral sclerosis. Some patients have most of their motor neuron disease affecting their speech and swallowing muscles (progressive bulbar palsy).

ALS can start with weakness in a hand; it can start with weakness in a leg; and, in some patients, it starts with weakness in the speech and swallowing muscles. Regardless of where it starts, it tends over time to gradually spread and involve other areas of the body. ALS is believed in those patients to run a steadily progressive course of gradual loss of muscle strength and function. The rate of progression of disease is extremely variable from patient to patient and hard to predict early on in the course of the disease. Some patients have a rapidly progressive disease course and do not survive for a year. Other patients have a slow disease course, with a gentle slope of loss of function, and survive for 20 or 30 years or more. The largest group of patients with this disorder has a disease course that runs somewhere between 2 and 5 years from the onset of symptoms. Roughly 20% of patients have a slow course of disease progression, allowing survival beyond 5 years, and 10% of ALS patients have a disease course lasting more than 10 years (most patients in the end course of the disease have difficulty with breathing and swallowing). Other than muscle cramps, which are fairly common (and can be treated with quinine), ALS is not painful. ALS does not cause loss of sensations, vision problems, and usually does not cause bladder or bowel problems. Importantly, ALS does not typically affect thinking or memory (although occasional patients may have an associated frontal lobe dementia).

For most patients, the cause of ALS is unknown. For about 5% to 10% of patients, the cause is known to be genetic in that the disease runs in families, occurring in members of every generation. About one fifth of the patients with the genetic or familial form of ALS have abnormal DNA involving the gene that codes for an enzyme, superoxide dismutase.

Management requires a comprehensive multidisciplinary team approach to addressing the various functional limitations imposed by the disease (Box 4).

Box 4. Therapy for amyotrophic lateral sclerosis

Symptomatic treatment
- Muscle cramps: Quinine (260 mg), one tablet each evening, is safe and also effective. If that does not work, gabapentin at low doses, carbamazepine, or vitamin E can be effective.
- Fasciculations: Most patients are not bothered by their muscle twitches in the disease, but if the twitches are disturbing the patient, gabapentin or carbamazepine may help.
- Stiffness or spasticity: There are several medications that can be helpful in reducing some of the tightness and spasticity that occurs with upper motor neuron disease, including baclofen, tizanidine, and diazepam.
- Frequent laughing and crying (pseudo-bulbar affect): Amitriptyline, fluoxetine, sertraline, and, more recently, dextromethorphan and quinidine, can be effective.
- Foot drop (or the foot dangles or toes catch on the ground): ankle-foot orthosis.
- Wrist drop or significant weakness in the forearm or hand: Wrist splint.
- Trouble walking or sitting: Patients may benefit by working with a good physical therapist over time. Aids in walking include exercises, canes (several different types), rolling walkers, and, if the legs are weak enough, some type of wheelchair. There are lightweight manual wheelchairs, but some patients benefit from motorized scooters or motorized wheelchairs. A good physical therapist can help get the patient get around optimally.
- Difficulty doing things with hands, such as grasping items, getting dressed, preparing meals, typing at a keyboard, and turning a car ignition: Patients benefit by working with a good occupational therapist on a long-term basis. The occupational therapist may recommend splints, exercises, and stretching as

well as suggestions for how to get the optimal function out of a weak hand or arm. In addition, occupational therapists have a wide variety of aids that can make it easy to fasten fasteners and accomplish other activities that may be difficult if the hands are weak.

- Dysarthria: A good speech therapist can be helpful. There are some techniques to improve communication; if speech and writing become too limited, there are various electronic speech devices that allow satisfactory exchange of communication.
- Dysphagia: This is a common problem in ALS. Patients may find that swallowing is a slow process taking so much time that they lose weight from lack of nutrition. Also, some patients choke with swallowing, which poses serious risk. The speech therapist typically serves as a "swallowing therapist" and can provide tips on what types of foods and liquids the patient should use, suggest simple techniques to improve the efficiency and safety of swallowing (such as the chin tuck), and monitor the patient's progress. If swallowing is difficult to the point that the patient is losing weight from malnutrition or is choking excessively, placement of a feeding tube directly into the stomach (PEG tube) may be beneficial.
- Drooling and difficulty handling oral secretions: This is a vexing problem for many patients. Medications such as glycopyrrolate, atropine, amitriptyline, or an ipratropium bromide spray can reduce the amount of saliva produced in the mouth, which can be helpful. Also, a suction machine in the home can be helpful, if needed. If the patient suffers from excessive oral secretions, and suggested measures are ineffective, a tracheostomy should be considered as a comfort measure. Botox of the parotid glands may be tried.
- Respiratory involvement: This is not only common but often overlooked until late. Low threshold for biPap and a formal pulmonary evaluation may be needed.
- The need for a team of multiple specialists: Some patients benefit not only from seeing a pulmonologist for breathing trouble and a gastroenterologist for swallowing trouble, but also from seeing a specialist in physical medicine and rehabilitation (PM&R). The PM&R physician is in the ideal position to evaluate the patient's overall functional status and orchestrate the optimal management program. Because many patients have a wide variety of symptomatic problems and need to see various specialists, it is helpful to have a multidisciplinary ALS clinic system in which patients can in

the same half-day see not only their neurologist but also a physical medicine and rehabilitation physician, social service professional, physical therapist, occupational therapist, and nursing support services, providing the patient access to input from multiple experts.

Treating the underlying disease

To treat the underlying loss of motor neurons in this disease, the only drug that has been shown to be of some benefit as of this writing is riluzole 50 mg twice daily. Riluzole inhibits release of glutamate, and ostensibly reduces excitotoxicity. Studies indicate that taking the drug prolongs survival by about 2 to 3 months on average. The drug does not cure the disease or halt its progression, so it is difficult to see its effect on a patient's course. But patients who take the drug may be getting a benefit at slowing down the disease. All other medical therapies are unproven at this juncture.

Case 4: Kennedy's Disease

This 30-year-old man presented with 10 years of slowly progressive trouble walking and going up and down stairs (Fig. 4). His course has been slowly progressive and painless. He denies sensory loss. The family history is notable for a similar condition in his brother and also his maternal grandfather. Exam shows symmetrical atrophy in the limbs with fasciculations.

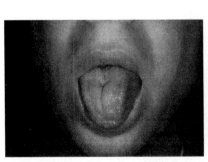
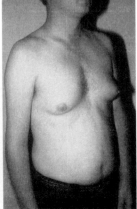

Fig. 4. Kennedy's disease patient.

He has reduced muscle stretch reflexes throughout. Sensation is normal. The tongue is atrophic with fasciculations. The exam is as shown in the figure. What is the diagnosis, appropriate workup, and prognosis?

Discussion

The patient's bulbar and proximal muscle weakness with fasciculations is indicative of bulbar onset ALS. On examination the following day in the clinic, the patient has absent reflexes and is otherwise as described above. MRI of the cervical spine shows no significant cord or nerve root compression. Nerve conduction studies show essentially normal responses. Needle EMG shows increased insertional activity, with large motor units in all proximal muscles. Though suggestive of bulbar onset ALS, the gynecomastia, pure lower motor neuron disorder, and positive family history suggest x-linked bulbospinal muscular atrophy or Kennedy's disease. Kennedy's disease has a much slower clinical course than ALS, with many patients having a normal life expectancy. The disorder is due to a defect in the androgen receptor gene (and the gene test is commercially available).

Case 5: Myotonic Dystrophy

This 37-year-old man presented to the clinic with his mother complaining of 5 years of slowly progressive difficulty using the hands (Fig. 5). The patient appears unconcerned and apathetic to the visit; however, his mother reports he has been having difficulty holding on to objects. While eliciting the family history, the patient's mother states he looks just like his father, who died at the age of 45 from a sudden cardiac arrhythmia.

The examination shows features revealed in the picture with prominent frontal balding, mild ptosis, and temporalis muscle wasting. There is

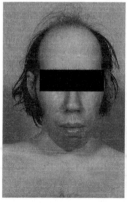
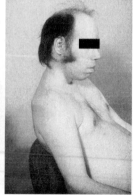
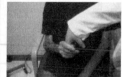

Fig. 5. Myotonic dystrophy patient.

weakness and atrophy of the facial, sternocleidomastoid, and hand muscles. Strength is reduced at 4/5, being weaker distally than proximally. What is the diagnosis, appropriate workup, and management?

Discussion

Myotonic dystrophy often presents with slow progressive symptoms and signs of predominantly distal muscle weakness [10,11]. This patient exhibits the characteristic myotonic dystrophy facies with bitemporal wasting, resulting in a long, lean face. Weakness is significant in the sternocleidomastoid muscle, and distal greater than proximal muscles with atrophy, resulting in weakness of the hands or foot drop. Myotonia, a characteristic feature of this disorder, may manifest with slow release from a forceful grip, muscle contraction after tapping with a reflex hammer (percussion myotonia), and myotonic discharges on EMG needle exam. Gene testing is commercially available. Myotonic dystrophy can present at any age from childhood to the elderly. In general, the age of onset and severity of symptoms are related to the length of trinucleotide repeat expansion. Severe cases present at birth with a floppy baby (typically displaying a tented mouth). Babies will not display EMG nor clinical myotonia, and the best clinical test is to simply examine the child's mother. Myotonic dystrophy is probably the most common of the muscular dystrophies that present in adulthood. It is one of the few diagnoses that physicians cannot afford to miss for several reasons. It is autosomal dominant, and so when one patient is diagnosed there is an entire family of potentially affected individuals. Second, as indicated by this patient's apathy toward his own symptoms, few patients present with early symptoms. Most patients with this condition are not aware that they are affected. Last, and most important, this disorder is a true systemic disease. Beyond muscle weakness, patients commonly have cardiac rhythm disturbance (which can be fatal but is often treatable), obstructive sleep apnea, central sleep apnea, dysphagia, gastrointestinal problems (such as gall bladder disease), endocrinopathy (such as diabetes), learning disabilities, cataracts, and others.

Management

Patients are often jointly managed in muscular dystrophy clinics as well as cardiology clinics with yearly ECG to monitor arrhythmias, as roughly 5% require pacemakers during their lifetime. Management in a Muscular Dystrophy Association clinic can facilitate ankle-foot orthosis and hand splint fitting as well as assist with other devices as patients progressively get weaker. Patients should also receive occasional sleep studies as they frequently suffer from nocturnal hypoventilation as a result of diaphragmatic weakness. This may improve with bilevel positive airway pressure (BiPAP) therapy. Genetic counseling is indicated.

Case 6: Myotonia Congenita

This 25-year-old man presented with symptoms dating back to childhood of intermittent stiffness and slowness of walking, running, and using his arms and hands. He states that his hands tend to cramp up on him at work (he manages a grocery store). His cramps are painless. The stiffness appears to improve the more active he is through the day. His stiffness is also more problematic in cold weather. Since childhood he has been considered to have a muscular body (even though he does not routinely workout). On examination (Fig. 6), the patient has a muscular build and has normal strength and reflexes. Upon checking grip strength he is slow to relax and release his grasp. Percussion of the thenar muscles results in tensing up of the muscle (percussion myotonia). His sister (See Fig. 6; Fig. 7) also is muscular and has similar symptoms of lifelong stiffness. They have several other relatives with similar symptoms. What is the diagnosis and appropriate workup?

Discussion

This patient has myotonia congenita, a generally benign myotonic disorder. The most common form is a hereditary disorder of the chloride channel gene inherited in autosomal dominant fashion. The presence of near-continuous muscle contraction results in muscle hypertrophy. The stiffness is exacerbated by cold temperatures or rest, and improves with heat and exercise. Muscle enzymes and biopsy are usually normal. EMG shows prominent myotonic discharges but normal voluntary motor units. The differential

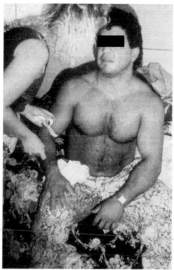
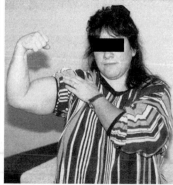

Fig. 6. Twenty-five-year-old man with lifelong muscle stiffness. Exam shows prominent muscularity.

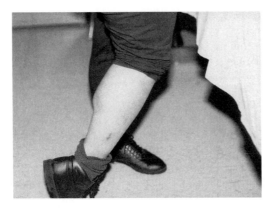

Fig. 7. Twenty-seven-year-old sister of the patient with similar symptoms.

diagnosis includes myotonic dystrophy distinguished on the basis of progressive weakness and the myriad of other systemic complications. Paramyotonia congenita can also presents in infancy with muscle stiffness triggered by cold and hypertrophy. In paramyotonia congenita, however, stiffness is aggravated by repeated use of the muscle (thus paradoxical) as well frank muscle weakness upon exposure to cold. For patients with severe symptoms of myotonia congenita drug therapy with membrane stabilizers, such as carbamazepine, phenytoin, mexiletine, can result in symptomatic improvement.

Case 7: Fascioscapulohumoral Muscular Dystrophy

This 60-year-old man presented with 10 years of slowly progressive difficulty using his arms over his head (Fig. 8). He recalls that his mother

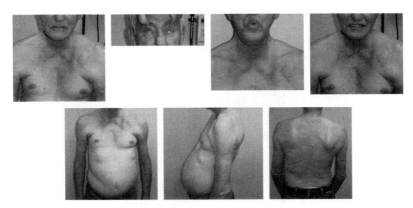

Fig. 8. Fascioscapulohumoral (FSH) muscular dystrophy patient. Pectoral folds, scapular winging, and atrophy of the humoral muscles. The man cannot whistle and has weakness of the orbicularis oculi (bifacial weakness).

and brother have experienced somewhat similar symptoms with shoulder weakness. Exam is shown in the photos. He has 4/5 strength in the upper arms, scapular winging, and also bifacial weakness. Sensation and reflexes are normal. Muscle enzymes are mildly elevated. What is the best diagnosis?

Discussion

The patient has fascioscapulohumoral muscular dystrophy (FSH dystrophy), which is among the most common of adult-onset muscular dystrophies. The condition is inherited as an autosomal dominant disorder. Most patients have the onset of symptoms in their late teenage years. Unlike myotonic dystrophy and the dystrophinopathies, patients typically do not have cardiac or other systemic complications, and life expectancy is unaffected. Often the clinical manifestations are mild and cosmetic.

Case 8: Becker's Dystrophy

This 25-year-old man presented with 10 to 15 years of gradual progressive difficulty with walking, running, and going up and down stairs (Fig. 9). He recently was evaluated for syncope and has been told that he has a cardiomyopathy. The exam shows a waddling gait and 4/5 proximal weakness. His muscle enzymes are elevated. The other important exam findings can be observed in the figure.

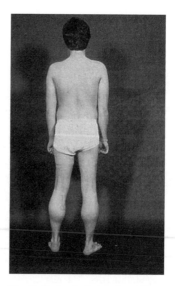

Fig. 9. Becker's dystrophy patient.

Discussion

The presence of calf muscle hypertrophy in the setting of years of progressive proximal weakness should raise the question of muscular dystrophy and more specifically a dystrophinopathy. The most common disorder of dystrophin is Duchenne dystrophy, affecting boys with presentation around age 5, weakness sufficient to require a wheelchair around age 10, and survival most often limited by diaphragm weakness around age 20. These boys typically have calf muscle hypertrophy. The diagnosis can be confirmed in 80% with a gene test looking for a mutation involving the dystrophin gene (and the remaining patients with a muscle biopsy showing scant or no dystrophin). Corticosteroids can slow down the relentless progression of weakness to a limited extent. Most of the management is multidisciplinary supportive management, including evaluation of respiratory and in teenage years cardiac status. Cardiomyopathy is fairly common. As the patient above is 25 years old and still walking, he does not have Duchenne dystrophy. A partial or milder dystrophinopathy is referred to as Becker's dystrophy. These patients have similar genetic defects of the dystrophin gene but have sufficient dystrophin in muscle to allow for a slower clinical course. Often they present with cardiac problems as in the patient above.

Case 9: Corticosteroid Myopathy

This 35-year-old woman presented with 6 months of progressive difficulty getting up from a chair and going up and down stairs (Fig. 10). She has noted a 50-pound weight gain during this time. In her exam, she appears puffy, has cataracts, is hypertensive, and bruises easily, as shown in the photos. She has symmetrical proximal weakness in the arms and legs at 4/5. Sensation and reflex exam are normal. She walks with a waddling gait.

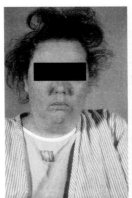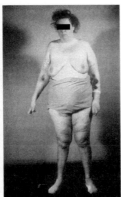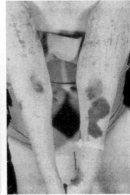

Fig. 10. Corticosteroid myopathy patient.

Muscle enzymes and EMG are normal. What is the diagnosis and how do you confirm your suspicion?

Discussion

The patient appears to be Cushingoid, and with the presence of proximal weakness the diagnosis is corticosteroid myopathy. Most such patients have iatrogenic disease, but in this patient she was not taking any corticosteroid medication. Her Cushing syndrome is the result of an adrenal tumor. Patients with corticosteroid myopathy typically have other clinical manifestations of Cushing syndrome. This myopathy is one of the few in which muscle enzymes are never elevated. Such patients typically have a normal or nonspecifically mildly abnormal EMG and muscle biopsy (therefore, no muscle biopsy was performed in this patient). The best diagnostic test in patients who are developing proximal weakness on corticosteroid medication is to decrease their dosage and observe for clinical improvement in strength over weeks to months.

Case 10: Inflammatory Myopathy

This 60-year-old woman presented with a 6-month history of gradual progressive difficulty going up and down stairs, rising from a chair, and using her arms over her head (Fig. 11). In the past 2 months she has developed a skin rash on the face and hands. Sensation and reflexes are normal. Proximal strength is reduced to 4/5. Muscle enzymes are elevated. What is the diagnosis?

Discussion

There are three common forms of myositis—polymyositis, dermatomyositis, and inclusion body myositis (IBM). They each account for roughly one third of subacute or chronic myositis [7–9]. Note that viral myositis is typically transient, lasting only a week or two. Often, by the time testing is

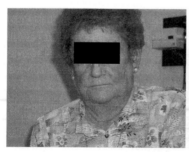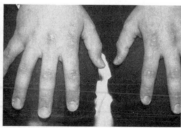

Fig. 11. Myositis patient.

arranged, the patient's symptoms have resolved. Except for the skin lesions, polymyositis and dermatomyositis are similar in their clinical presentation—proximal weakness in the neck flexors/extensors, shoulders, and hips. These patients often complain of loss of a specific function, such as trouble rising from a chair or climbing stairs, rather than overall weakness. And most myositis patients have little or no pain. Although most clinicians are taught that that polymyositis is the most common inflammatory myopathy, it may be one of the least common. One should be cautious about making this diagnosis. The diagnosis is often confused with mixed connective tissue diseases and various forms of muscular dystrophy.

The examination shows symmetrical proximal weakness, normal sensation, preserved reflexes, and not much cranial weakness except for dysphagia, which is seen in about 25% of patients. Though uncommon, patients with acute severe myositis may have diaphragm involvement and respiratory failure. The skin lesions in dermatomyositis include heliotrope rash (violet rash on the eyelids, named after the heliotrope plant. The flowers face the sunlight in the morning and follow the sun across the sky as the day progresses, thus the name of heliotrope), red scaly lesions on the knuckles, elbows, knees, butterfly rash on the face, rash on the sun-exposed regions of the head/neck/trunk, and periungual edema.

Systemic manifestations of dermato- and polymyositis can include fatigue, weight loss, arthralgias, and fever. Cardiac involvement can lead to arrhythmia, heart block, or congestive failure. Interstitial lung fibrosis can lead to various respiratory problems. Dysphagia and other GI motility abnormalities may occur. About 25% of older patients with dermatomyositis will have an associated malignancy.

Inclusion body myositis should be suspected in patients with years of slowly progressive weakness, especially with prominent involvement of quadriceps and distal finger flexor muscles. IBM patients can also develop substantial dysphagia and bifacial weakness. EMG needle exam tends to show profuse fibrillation. Immunosuppressive treatment is typically ineffective in IBM.

Laboratory Findings

Laboratory findings in dermatomyositis/polymyositis include elevated creatine kinase (CK) in 90% of patients. EMG is abnormal in 90%, indicating the presence of a myopathy; fibrillation suggests an active component and may help distinguish inclusion body myositis as well as help select the muscle to biopsy. Muscle biopsy should distinguish the three common forms of inflammatory myopathy (and help diagnose the uncommon forms as well):

- Polymyositis: muscle fiber necrosis, cellular infiltration
- Dermatomyositis: vasculopathy, vasculitis, perifascicular atrophy

- Inclusion body myositis: inflammation and rimmed vacuoles on H&E, oil red O, EM shows filamentous inclusions

Case 11: Inclusion Body Myositis

This 59-year-old man presented with a 5- to 6-year history of trouble holding objects and getting out of chairs. He was formerly a home painter but had to accept an early retirement because of difficulty holding his paint cans and brushes. He also noticed a progressive difficulty climbing ladders and getting out of chairs. The examination shows mild generalized weakness with marked weakness of the bilateral finger flexors, quadriceps, and foot dorsiflexors. There is atrophy of the quadriceps, and reflexes are absent or diminished throughout. Muscle enzymes are mildly elevated. What is the diagnosis, appropriate workup, and management?

Discussion

The patient has a painless progressive muscle weakness more pronounced in the distal muscles. This insidious onset of weakness of both proximal and distal muscles is suggestive of inclusion body myositis (IBM), considered be the most common inflammatory myopathy in individuals older than age 50. Prominent distal weakness is a frequent finding especially of the distal finger flexors. Atrophy of quadriceps muscles and diminished reflexes are also common. Many patients are misdiagnosed as a result of the insidious progression and similarities to polymyositis or motor neuron disease. CK levels are either normal or only mildly elevated. EMG often shows evidence for a chronic myopathy with an active component (fibrillation) and at times shows some mild neurogenic features. Muscle biopsy shows inflammatory infiltrates, rimmed vacuoles, and intranuclear and cytoplasmic inclusions. The condition progresses at an extremely slow rate (years and at time decades) compared with dermatomyositis and polymyositis, in which progression is typically over several months. One should be leery of a diagnosis of chronic polymyositis, as many such patients turn out on further review to have IBM.

Management

Management of IBM is mainly symptomatic. Though it shares the presence of inflammatory infiltrates with the other idiopathic inflammatory myopathies, dermatomyositis and polymyositis, it does not share the responsiveness to corticosteroids or other immunotherapy. Knowing the lack of responsiveness to immunotherapy should influence decision-making regarding use of long-term corticosteroids or other potentially hazardous options. Patients are supported with physical and occupational therapy and equipment for adaptation. Speech and swallowing therapy and pulmonary evaluation for hypoventilation is useful as patients often eventually develop bulbar or respiratory weakness.

Case 12: McArdle's Disease

This 22-year-old man presented to the emergency department. A fire broke out at his workplace and he sprinted 40 yards to grab a fire extinguisher and sprinted back to the fire but en route his leg and back muscles became painfully tight and he fell to the ground. In the emergency room he had symmetrical leg weakness at 4/5 with swollen and painful muscles if the legs, shoulders, and back. His CK was elevated to 90,000. He was admitted for hydration and monitoring for renal failure. Over several days his weakness and muscle pain gradually resolved, and 2 weeks later his clinical exam and CK were normal. His past history is notable for quitting the football team in high school for several similar though less severe episodes. What is your diagnosis?

Discussion

The patient has exercise-induced rhabdomyoloyis, raising the question of a metabolic myopathy. From the diagnostic standpoint, patients with glycolytic enzyme defects tend to have exercise-induced contractures—a painful muscle contraction that is electrically silent. It differs from a true muscle cramp, which is electrically active. A screening test for the glycolytic enzyme defects is the ischemic exercise test. The forearm ischemic exercise test is performed as follows: An IV is placed in the anticubital fossa or in the forearm and the baseline venous lactate and ammonia level are obtained, then the patient has a blood pressure cuff raised above the systolic level and for 1 minute the patient is asked to grip a dynamometer repeatedly as intensely as possible. After 1 minute, the blood pressure cuff is released and venous lactate and ammonia levels are checked immediately and then at 1, 2, 4, 6, 10, and 20 minutes following exercise. Normally, both the lactate and ammonia levels will rise within several minutes. In a patient with no rise in either lactate or ammonia, the test result should be considered inconclusive and perhaps exercise was inadequate. In patients with phosphorylase deficiency or with one of the other glycolytic enzyme abnormalities, the ammonia level rises appropriately but the lactate level does not (ie, the ammonia level is the control). On the occasion that the serum lactate rises normally but the ammonia does not, one should consider myoadenylate deaminase deficiency. Further diagnostic options include gene testing as well as muscle biopsy staining for phoshorylase.

This patient has phophorylase deficiency (McArdle's disease) [12]. Most patients learn to avoid exercise that requires intense anaerobic metabolism. The breakdown of glycogen early in exercise is central to energy metabolism in muscles. In patients with phosphorylase deficiency (McArdle's disease), the glycolytic enzyme defect blocks glycogenolysis in muscles, which limits exercise tolerance and in the first few minutes of intense exercise tends to lead to severe symptoms of muscle pain, weakness, and rhabdomyolysis.

A recent study by Vissing and Haller [13] reports results of a single-blind randomized placebo-controlled crossover study of 12 patients with phosphorylase deficiency who drank a 75-g sucrose load about a half hour before 15 minutes of a stationary bicycle workout. The results were positive, suggesting that sucrose 75 g a half hour before exercise may markedly improve exercise tolerance in patients with phosphorylase deficiency, improve the patient's exercise capacity and sense of well-being, and potentially protect against acute exercise-induced rhabdomyolysis.

Case 13: Mitochondrial Myopathy

This 40-year-old woman presented with 15 years of slowly progressive droopy eyelids and double vision (Fig. 12). Though she has carried a diagnosis of myasthenia gravis, she denies any fluctuation in her symptoms throughout the day. She has for the past 2 years developed mild dysphagia. She has been treated with pyridostigmine and also with prednisone with no benefit. Past edrophonium chloride test, repetitive stimulation, and acetylcholine receptor antibody studies have been normal. Creatine kinase is mildly elevated at 290, and EMG needle exam is normal. The exam is shown in Fig. 12. What is the diagnosis and appropriate diagnostic test?

Discussion

The patient has a chronic progressive external ophthalmoplegia typical for mitochondrial myopathy. Any patient with a slow progressive ophthalmoplegia should be considered for a mitochondrial disorder. Some mitochondrial disorders are associated with cardiomyopathy, short stature, scoliosis, or retinitis pigmentosa (Kearns-Sayre syndrome), whereas others have symptoms limited to ophthalmoplegia . Specialists often refer to CPEO as "ragged red fiber disease" or "ophthalmoplegia plus" (Fig. 13). Patients typically experience a slow progressive course of symmetrical weakness. Management is supportive with attention to cardiac function and management of dysphagia.

Case 14: Hypothyroidism

This 57-year-old man presented with an 8-month history of progressive difficulty getting up from a chair and going up and down stairs (Fig. 14). He has noted a 60-pound weight gain during this time. He is chilly most

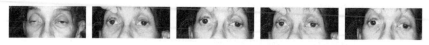

Fig. 12. Nonfluctuating ptosis. Patient is looking up, down, right, and left (severe ophthalmoparesis).

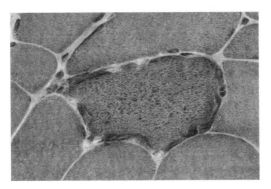

Fig. 13. Muscle biopsy. Gomari trichrome stain showing "ragged red fiber" typical for mitochondrial myopathy.

of the time. Exam shows proximal weakness at 4/5 with normal sensation. The ankle jerks are slow in the relaxation phase. Face as shown in the photo appears puffy with sallow complexion and thinning of the lateral third of the eyebrow. Cholesterol is elevated, and CK is 600. What is your diagnosis?

Discussion

This patient is hypothyroid and has a related myopathy. Many hypothyroid patients have nonspecific fatigue or cramping, aching, and muscles soreness without actual weakness. Elevated muscle enzymes are common in hypothyroidism, even in the absence of weakness. As with this patient, hypothyroidism can cause a frank myopathy with severe proximal weakness. This patient returned to normal about 6 months after initiation of replacement therapy.

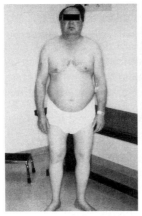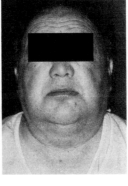

Fig. 14. Hypothyroid patient.

Case 15: Statin Myopathy

A 52-year-old man presented with 2 weeks of severe muscle pain most prominent in the legs. The symptoms began soon after the patient was seen by his primary care physician for a physical and routine blood work, which was normal except for only moderately elevated LDL cholesterol. On examination the patient exhibits mild weakness of the bilateral proximal lower extremities. He notes that his urine has been a dark tealike color over the last day. Lab work performed in the office shows a CK of about 10,000 u/l. What is the diagnosis, appropriate workup, and management?

Discussion

Symptoms of statin myopathy include severe myalgia, weakness, and CK of greater than 10 times the upper limit of normal. Myoglobinuria is of concern in a patient who recently started a HMG-CoA reductase inhibitor (statin) for a statin-associated myopathy. Persistent myalgia is a known side effect to the category of drugs known as statins, affecting up to 5% of patients. Less common in the broad spectrum of this condition is the myositis and rhabdomyolysis that is potentially life-threatening, which appears to be affecting this patient. Factors that appear to influence the incidence of symptomatic myalgia include dose, body size, renal insufficiency, hepatic disease, hypothyroidism, age, diabetes, and concomitant use of other drugs affecting cytochrome P-450 (CYP) 3A4 pathway. Most clinically significant myositis is associated with elevation of CK.

Treatment

In cases with myositis and rhabdomyolysis, immediate withdrawal of statin is indicated. Patients with myalgia and CK elevation also should discontinue the medication and consider an alternate agent. Care should be taken to ensure the CK is not falsely elevated, as statin therapy magnifies the normal increase in CK seen after strenuous exercise. Asymptomatic patients with elevated CK may continue on therapy as long as CK does not rise to greater than 10 times upper limit of normal. Patients with myalgia without elevated CK may also continue on therapy as long as symptoms are tolerable. Rare cases where myalgia and CK elevation persist after withdrawal of statin therapy should prompt a workup for other causes that may have been unmasked, such as hypothyroidism, polymyalgia rheumatica, or temporal arteritis.

Case 16: Myasthenia Gravis

This uninsured monster presented to the office with several months of symptoms of weakness. As is typical with many patients these days, he brings in a 195-page book of his symptoms and past medical history and insists that the physicians read it to better understand his problem.

The monster has symptoms of fatigable weakness of the limbs as well as dysphonia (Box 5) [14]. The photos indicate that he has fluctuating ptosis (Fig. 15) [15]. The diagnosis must then be myasthenia gravis (MG). This case was shared with colleagues who felt that the diagnosis was unlikely in part because the monster is so unique and there is no underlying explanation for why he might develop MG. But there is an explanation. In most patients, the cause of autoimmune MG is unknown. However, there are three iatrogenic causes for autoimmune MG. D-penicillamine (used in the treatment of Wilson's disease and rheumatoid arthritis) and alfa-interferon therapy are both capable of inducing MG. In addition, bone marrow transplantation is associated with the development of MG as part of the chronic graft versus host disease. And who would be the ultimate candidate for a chronic graft versus host disease? This monster was assembled by Dr. Frankenstein from a broad variety of donors. This is without doubt the mother of all transplant patients. If there is anyone prone to getting a chronic graft versus host disease, it would be this monster.

Box 5. Patient's reported symptoms

"But this was a luxury of sensation that could not endure; I became fatigued with excess of bodily exertion and sank on the damp grass in the sick impotence of despair. There was none among the myriads of men that existed who would pity or assist me; and should I feel kindness towards my enemies? No; from that moment I declared everlasting war against the species, and more than all, against him who had formed me and sent me forth to this insupportable misery.

"These thoughts exhilarated me and led me to apply with fresh ardour to the acquiring the art of language. My organs were indeed harsh, but supple;

"My heart beat quick; this was the hour and moment of trial, which would decide my hopes or realize my fears. The servants were gone to a neighbouring fair. All was silent in and around the cottage; it was an excellent opportunity; yet , when I proceeded to execute my plan, my limbs failed me and I sank to the ground. Again I rose, and exerting all the firmness of which I was master, removed the planks which I had placed before my hovel to conceal my retreat. The fresh air revived me, and with renewed determination I approached the door of their cottage."

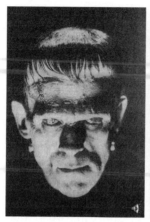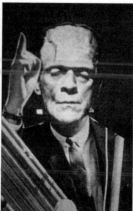

Fig. 15. The monster demonstrates ptosis (right eye 50% and left eye 75%). The ptosis is 100% in both eyes. (© Universal Studios; used with permission.)

Management

Serology for acetylcholine receptor antibodies and chest imaging for thymoma were obtained. Because of the severity of symptoms, thymectomy was performed on this patient. The monster was lost to follow-up several months later, and thus long-term outcome data are not available.

References

[1] Pascuzzi RM. Pearls and pitfalls in the diagnosis and management of neuromuscular junction disorders. Semin Neurol 2001;21:425–40.
[2] Meriggioli MN, Sanders DB. Myasthenia gravis: diagnosis. Semin Neurol 2004;24(1):31–9.
[3] Saperstein DS, Barohn RJ. Management of myasthenia gravis. Semin Neurol 2004;24(1): 41–8.
[4] Newsom-Davis J. Therapy in myasthenia gravis and Lambert-Eaton myasthenic syndrome. Semin Neurol 2003;23:191–8.
[5] Mareska M, Gutmann L. Lambert-Eaton myasthenic syndrome. Semin Neurol 2004;24: 149–53.
[6] Pascuzzi RM. ALS, motor neuron disease, and related disorders: a personal approach to diagnosis and management. Semin Neurol 2002;22:75–87.
[7] Kissel JT. Misunderstanding, misperceptions, and mistakes in the management of the myopathies. Semin Neurol 2002;22:41–51.
[8] Donofrio PD. Immunotherapy of idiopathic inflammatory neuropathies. Muscle Nerve 2003;28:273–92.
[9] Dalakas MC. Therapeutic approaches in patients with inflammatory myopathies. Semin Neurol 2003;23:199–206.
[10] Schoser BG, Ricker K, Schneider-Gold C, Hengstenberg C, Durre J, Bultmann B, et al. Sudden cardiac death in myotonic dystrophy type 2. Neurology 2004;63:2402–4.
[11] Groh WJ, Lowe MR, Simmons Z, Bhakta D, Pascuzzi RM. Familial clustering of muscular and cardiac involvement in myotonic dystrophy type 1. Muscle Nerve 2005;31: 719–24.

[12] Sinnreich M, Sorenson EJ, Klein CJ. Neurologic course, endocrine dysfunction and triplet repeat size in spinal bulbar muscular atrophy. Can J Neurol Sci 2004;31:378–82.

[13] Vissing J, Haller RG. The effect of oral sucrose on exercise tolerance in patients with McArdle's disease. New Engl J Med 2003;349(26):2503.

[14] Shelley M. Frankenstein. Bantam Classics.

[15] Pascuzzi RM. Historical notes: pearls and pitfalls in the horror cinema. Semin Neurol 1998; 18:267–73.

ELSEVIER
SAUNDERS

Neurol Clin 24 (2006) 267–289

NEUROLOGIC
CLINICS

Sleep Disorders: Case Studies

Mark W. Mahowald, MD[a,b,*],
Michel A. Cramer Bornemann, MD[a,b]

[a]Minnesota Regional Sleep Disorders Center, Hennepin County Medical Center,
701 Park Avenue, Minneapolis, MN 55415, USA
[b]Department of Neurology, University of Minnesota Medical School, 420 Delaware Street SE,
Minneapolis, MN 55455, USA

Case 1: "Passing-Out" Spells

A 23-year-old man was referred to the sleep clinic for evaluation of a 3-year history of progressively severe, inappropriate excessive daytime sleepiness (EDS). He stated: "I can fall asleep any time, anywhere, any place." He had fallen asleep during noisy social events and had even fallen asleep standing up. He also complained of "short faints," which were described as episodes of muscle weakness, particularly involving the knees, triggered by any type of emotion. He stated: "With laughter, I go out." His first episode of weakness occurred when he was working as a busboy; he dropped an entire tray of dishes he was carrying when he laughed at a joke. He has hypnagogic hallucinations, described as perceiving a "presence in my room" once weekly. There was no history of sleep paralysis. His past history was remarkable for remote head injuries without neurologic sequellae. The physical examination was normal.

Questions

What Is the Differential Diagnosis?

The practical differential diagnosis of EDS is short: volitional sleep deprivation, obstructive sleep apnea, narcolepsy, or idiopathic CNS hypersomnia. In this case, narcolepsy would be likely, in view of a history suggestive of cataplexy.

---

* Corresponding author. Minnesota Regional Sleep Disorders Center, Hennepin County Medical Center, 701 Park Avenue, Minneapolis, MN 55415, USA.
  E-mail address: mahow002@umn.edu (M.W. Mahowald).

0733-8619/06/$ - see front matter © 2006 Elsevier Inc. All rights reserved.
doi:10.1016/j.ncl.2006.01.010

What Studies Should Be Performed?

A formal polysomnogram (PSG) should be performed to evaluate the quality and quantity of sleep the night before a multiple sleep latency test (MSLT) is performed. The PSG would rule out other causes of EDS, such as obstructive sleep apnea. The MSLT is a standardized and well-validated measure of physiologic sleepiness. The MSLT is designed to quantitate sleepiness by measuring how quickly an individual falls asleep on sequential naps during the day and to identify the abnormal occurrence of sleep-onset REM (SOREM) during a nap. For each nap, the latency between lights out and sleep onset is recorded. Pathologic ranges of sleep latency have been carefully defined. A mean latency of 5 minutes or less indicates severe excessive sleepiness. The number of naps during which episodes of SOREM appears is also noted. Patients with narcolepsy often display REM sleep on two or more naps. REM sleep during daytime naps in nonnarcoleptics is uncommon. Many factors can affect sleep latency during the daytime: prior sleep deprivation, sleep continuity, age, time of day, physiological arousal before nap opportunities, meals, and medications [1]. From a technical standpoint, early termination of PSGs such that patients are not allowed to wake up spontaneously may contribute to sleep deprivation, resulting in false-positive MSLTs. Nonetheless, the MSLT is a most useful tool in quantifying daytime sleepiness and in differentiating the subjective complaints of sleepiness, tiredness, and fatigue.

This patient's formal PSG was unremarkable. The total sleep time was 343 minutes with a sleep efficiency of 95%. A urine toxicology screen was negative for recreational drugs. A multiple sleep latency test the following day revealed a mean sleep latency of 2.4 minutes, with REM sleep occurring on four of five naps. This confirmed the complaint of severe hypersomnia. The appearance of REM sleep on two or more naps is highly suggestive of narcolepsy. For perspective, a nonnarcoleptic would have to miss an entire night's sleep to obtain a similar mean sleep latency.

MSLTs may be falsely negative. Therefore, telling a patient that he or she does not have a sleep disorder because the MSLT is normal is similar to telling a patient with chest pain that the pain cannot be cardiac in origin because the ECG is normal. All sleep studies must be interpreted in light of the entire clinical picture.

What Is the Diagnosis?

The combination of a clinical history of EDS with cataplexy along with an MSLT that has short mean sleep latency and two episodes of SOREM confirms that diagnosis of narcolepsy. Narcolepsy is a frequent disorder, with a prevalence of 0.09%, affecting at least 250,000 Americans. There is a clear genetic component, with over 90% of individuals with narcolepsy carrying the HLA-DR2/DQ1 (under current nomenclature HLA-DR15 and HLA-DQ6) gene (found in less than 30% of the general population) [2]. This association is present in the different ethnic populations to varying degrees, and represents the highest disease-HLA linkage known in medicine. Clearly, there is a genetic component; however, that component is neither necessary nor sufficient to cause narcolepsy.

Hypocretin-1, also known as orexin, plays an important role in narcolepsy. Hypocretin-1 is a neuropeptide of hypothalamic origin. It appears that patients with narcolepsy have lost the hypocretin-producing cells, possibly via an immune-mediated mechanism [3]. Undetectable CSF levels of hypocretin-1 are specific for patients with narcolepsy who have cataplexy and who are HLA DQB1*0602 positive, and absent CSF hypocretin-1 levels have not been found in any other conditions that could be confused with narcolepsy [4].

EDS is the primary symptom of narcolepsy. Ancillary symptoms include the classic "narcolepsy triad" of cataplexy, hypnagogic hallucinations, and sleep paralysis. Cataplexy occurs in 65% to 70% of patients with narcolepsy and is the sudden loss of muscle tone, typically triggered by emotion, such as laughter, anger, excitement, delight, or surprise. In many people with narcolepsy, the hypersomnia precedes the appearance of the ancillary symptoms, often by decades. Clearly, the absence of a history of cataplexy does not rule out the diagnosis of narcolepsy. Sleep paralysis and hypnagogic (occurring at sleep onset) or hypnopompic (occurring at sleep offset) hallucinations are also common in narcolepsy, but may also occur in nonnarcoleptics, particularly in the setting of sleep deprivation.

The underlying pathophysiology of narcolepsy results in impaired control of the boundaries that normally separate the states of wakefulness from REM and NREM sleep. The total sleep time per 24 hours in people with narcolepsy is similar to that in those without narcolepsy [5]. However, the control of the onset/offset of REM and non-REM sleep is impaired. Moreover, there is a clear dissociation of various components of the individual wake and sleep states. Cataplexy and sleep paralysis simply represent the isolated and inappropriate intrusion or persistence of REM sleep related atonia (paralysis) into wakefulness. The hypnagogic or hypnopompic hallucinations are (REM sleep-related) dreams occurring during wakefulness [2].

How Should This Be Managed?

Stimulant medications, such as amphetamine-based agents, amphetamine salt derivatives, such as methylphenidate, and modafinil are used to treat hypersomnolence. Though modafinil alone is FDA approved in the treatment of EDS associated with narcolepsy, there is no evidence that any of these agents are more or less effective than the other. Furthermore, no pharmacokinetic studies have been performed, rendering stated "maximum doses" arbitrary and without scientific basis. Many practitioners will titrate the medications to maximally control the symptoms [6]. The abuse potential for these agents in the bona-fide patient populations for which they are therapeutic has been greatly overrated, as have the cardiovascular and psychiatric consequences [6–10].

Treatment of cataplexy includes tricyclic antidepressants, serotonin-specific reuptake inhibitors, and gamma-hydroxy butyrate [11–13]. Venlafaxine, which inhibits the reuptake of norepinephrine, serotonin, and to a lesser extent dopamine, is often effective [14].

Case 2: Idiopathic Central Nervous System Hypersomnia Initially Misdiagnosed as Obstructive Sleep Apnea

A 32-year-old married Caucasian man, employed as an operations manager, was referred to the sleep disorders center for a second opinion. Since adolescence he has suffered from severe excessive daytime sleepiness. Regardless of how much sleep he obtained at night, he routinely fell asleep during periods of inactivity and reduced environmental stimulation. This reduced his effectiveness at work and compromised his safety, as well as others, while driving. Twelve years ago he had a fall-asleep motor vehicle crash. He stated: "At times, I feel that there is nothing that I can do to stay awake, no matter what I try." He had a history of automatic behavior, but no cataplexy, sleep paralysis, or hypnagogic hallucinations. He was known to snore and also had observed respiratory pauses during sleep. A review of systems and his past medical history were otherwise unremarkable. On examination, he stood 5'10", carried a weight of 230 pounds, and had a corresponding body mass index of 33.

Four years earlier the patient had been evaluated at an outside sleep clinic for the same complaint of EDS and was found to have, at worst, mild sleep apnea (respiratory disturbance index of four events per hour). He was placed on a nasal continuous positive airway pressure (CPAP) device with which he was staunchly compliant—with no improvement in his daytime sleepiness.

Questions

What Is the Differential Diagnosis?

There are few causes of EDS. The most common is volitional sleep deprivation for social or economic reasons. In the absence of sleep deprivation, the only other common causes of EDS are obstructive sleep apnea, narcolepsy, or idiopathic CNS hypersomnia. Although he had a history of snoring and observed apnea, the initial sleep study revealed trivial sleep apnea—clearly insufficient to explain his long-standing complaint of severe EDS. This leaves either narcolepsy or idiopathic CNS hypersomnia.

What Diagnostic Tests Should Be Performed?

A repeat formal polysomnographic (PSG) study followed by a (MSLT) the next day would be indicated. The PSG again revealed trivial sleep apnea with an apnea-hypopnea index of seven events per hour associated with negligible hemoglobin oxygen desaturation. The total sleep time was 489 minutes with a sleep efficiency of 90%. The MSLT revealed a mean sleep latency of 1.1 minutes without any episodes of SOREM occurring on any of five naps.

What Is the Diagnosis?

The MSLT provides objective evidence of severe daytime sleepiness. (For perspective, a normal individual would have to have remained awake all night to obtain a similar mean latency value—this means that this patient feels all day, every day, the way those without this condition feel after being up all night). The diagnosis is either monosymptomatic narcolepsy (narcolepsy without the ancillary symptoms of cataplexy, sleep paralysis, or hypnagogic hallucinations) or idiopathic CNS hypersomnia. Many individuals with narcolepsy do not have ancillary symptoms initially, and some may never develop cataplexy. Idiopathic CNS hypersomnia (IHS) may represent a number of different conditions that present as unexplained EDS. This condition characterized by EDS in the absence of sleep deprivation or other identifiable abnormality during sleep, such as obstructive sleep apnea [15]. The pathophysiology is unknown.

The diagnosis may be suspected by the history of unexplained EDS in the absence of symptoms suggestive of obstructive sleep apnea, narcolepsy, or sleep deprivation. Formal studies are mandatory to confirm the absence of unsuspected sleep-related pathologies and to confirm the subjective complaint of EDS. Chronic sleep deprivation must be aggressively ruled out as an explanation for EDS. Severe chronic sleep deprivation may affect the MSLT for several days, despite ad-lib sleep [16]. It is anticipated that further study of CSF hypocretin levels will likely aid in the proper classification of patients with various forms of hypersomnia.

How Should This Be Treated?

The treatment of the EDS in idiopathic hypersomnia is identical to the treatment of sleepiness in narcolepsy—stimulant medications, including methylphenidate, methamphetamine, dextroamphetamine, or modafinil [15].

What Is the Moral of This Story?

Sleep studies must be interpreted in light of the entire clinical picture. Clearly, although this patient did have mild (and clinically insignificant) sleep apnea, the observed degree of apnea would in no way explain either the severity of either the subjective complaint or objective degree of sleepiness. He responded better to stimulant medication than to CPAP.

Case 3: Insomnia

A retired 69-year-old married man was referred to the sleep clinic for evaluation of long-standing insomnia. He reported that for many years he had difficulty falling asleep, and on some nights stated that he did not sleep at all. The insomnia worsened following a surgical procedure a few months before the clinic visit. He had been prescribed a number of benzodiazepine and nonbenzodiazepine sedative-hypnotic agents with little benefit. He took occasional naps but had no symptoms of true excessive daytime sleepiness. He admitted to some depression that he attributed to his wife's serious medical problems. He states that he retires between 9 and 9:30 pm, and may or may not sleep at all during the night.

Questions

What Is the Differential Diagnosis?

Insomnia is by far the most common of all sleep-related complaints, probably exceeded only by pain in frequency of complaints to primary care physicians. Like pain, insomnia is a constitutional symptom and not a single diagnostic entity. It may also be the presenting symptom of other primary sleep disorders. A clear understanding of the probable cause of insomnia in a given case is essential before rational and effective treatment can be made.

Contrary to popular opinion, insomnia is often not due to psychiatric or psychological problems. Although there are numerous studies indicating that patients with insomnia have coexisting psychiatric problems, the causality dilemma associating insomnia with psychiatric problems, such as depression, remains unresolved. There is growing evidence that insomnia initially not associated with psychiatric problems, if untreated, is a significant risk factor for the development of psychiatric disorders [17].

It is well established that insomniacs differ from noninsomniacs in their perception of having been awake or asleep. The perception of having been asleep is inexact even in normal subjects, and is even worse in patients complaining of insomnia, who tend to overestimate the sleep latency and underestimate the total sleep time. There is growing evidence that many insomniacs may be in a constant state of hyperarousal. Many are less sleepy during the day than noninsomniacs as measured by MSLT, and they also have an increase in metabolic rate across the 24-hour period [18]. It has been proposed that chronic insomniacs may suffer from a more general disorder of hyperarousal that may be responsible for the daytime symptoms and poor nocturnal sleep [19].

Insomnia is not defined by the total sleep time but, rather, by the inability to obtain sleep that is sufficiently long or "good enough" to result in feeling rested or restored the following day. The total sleep requirement ranges between 4 and 10 hours. Therefore, a 4-hour sleeper who awakens rested and restored does not have insomnia but rather is simply a "short sleeper." Conversely, a 10-hour sleeper may have insomnia despite obtaining 8 hours of sleep nightly. Insomnia is a constitutional symptom, like pain, fever, or weight loss, and not a disorder in and of itself. In general, the complaint of insomnia requires a search for the underlying cause. Medical, psychiatric, and psychological conditions are only a few of the myriad of factors that may cause or worsen insomnia. One must also remain mindful to other factors, including environmental triggers, undiagnosed sleep disorders, and drug-induced influences. The most likely diagnostic possibilities in this particular case are conditioned (psychophysiological) or sleep state misperception (paradoxical) insomnia [20].

What Is the Diagnostic Approach to Insomnia?

A careful history and physical examination should rule out obvious underlying medical or psychiatric problems. All drugs (prescription, supplements, or recreational) should be identified. Prolonged (2–3 weeks) sleep/wake diaries completed by the patient or observer may give an at-a-glance overview of wake/sleep patterns not obviously apparent by clinical history.

Analysis of sleep diaries may be insufficient to verify a tentative diagnosis in patients with reported insomnia or suspected wake/sleep cycle abnormalities. In such cases, definitive objective data may be obtained by actigraphy, a recently developed technique to record activity during wake and sleep that supplements the subjective sleep log. An actigraph is a small wrist-mounted device that records the activity plotted against time—usually for 1 to 3 weeks. When data collection has been completed, the information is transferred to a personal computer for software analysis with the output displayed as a graphic plot of activity versus time. There is direct correlation between the rest/activity recorded by the actigraph and the wake/sleep pattern as determined by polysomnography [21]. Indications for the use of actigraphy include insomnia, wake/sleep schedule disorders, and monitoring treatment process. Without actigraphy, it may be nearly impossible to objectively evaluate particularly bizarre sleep complaints (as in the case of a patient who claims to sleep only 1 or 2 hours per night). In such cases, actigraphy is mandatory to confirm or refute the perceived sleep pattern before a treatment plan can be developed.

Formal sleep studies are rarely indicated in the evaluation of insomnia complaints. Exceptions include (1) a history of unexplained EDS (patients with insomnia complain of fatigue or lack of energy but uncommonly experience true excessive daytime sleepiness), (2) the suspicion of a coexisting sleep disorder, such as obstructive sleep apnea, or (3) lack of response to aggressive management of the insomnia.

What Should Be Done in This Case?

In view of this patient's subjective report of frequent nights of absolutely no sleep, an actigraphic study would be invaluable to confirm or refute this history. Without actigraphy, the physician has no way of knowing whether this patient has severe insomnia or paradoxical insomnia. Figure 1 shows the actigraphic pattern. Simultaneously recorded subjective sleep diaries indicated that he perceived receiving little sleep. On three of the nights, he subjectively recorded absolutely no sleep at all. Clearly, he is obtaining nearly normal amounts of sleep every night, and yet perceives that he sleeps little, if at all. This confirms the clinical suspicion of sleep-state misperception (paradoxical) insomnia.

What Is the Management?

Though time-intensive, an open educational dialog concerning sleep patterns and requirements often provides the patient with the reassurance

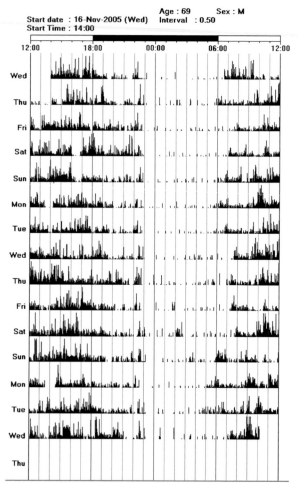

Fig. 1. Actigraphic study of paradoxical insomnia This is an actigraphic study of a patient who reports many nights of no sleep. The height of the bars indicates movement, which is highly correlated with wake/sleep. The actigraph indicates a clearly identifiable consolidated period of sleep, with sleep onset occurring at 11 pm and sleep offset occurring at 6 am to 8 am with rare nighttime awakenings. This supported the clinical diagnosis of sleep state misperception (paradoxical) insomnia.

needed to begin subjective improvement. Identifying and addressing potential dysfunctional attitudes and maladaptive coping strategies concerning sleep may also be of benefit. The actigraphic study results coupled with the history of no true excessive daytime sleepiness can be used to try to convince the patient that adequate sleep is being obtained.

Case 4: Disorder of Arousal

A 20-year-old college student is accompanied by his concerned and frightened parents to the sleep clinic because of a recent episode of dangerous activity arising from sleep five nights previously. He had fallen asleep at 1:30 am and awakened at 3 am to discover that he had shattered a window next to his bed and was lying in the glass shards on his bed, bleeding profusely from his wrist, knees, and nose. These injuries required sutures (Fig. 2). He had been sleep-deprived before this episode. Recreational drugs or alcohol were not involved.

His history of complex behaviors arising from sleep dates back to childhood. Once when staying at a cabin, he ran out into the street believing he was being chased. On another occasion, he had walked up to the railing of a boat and needed to be guided back to his bunk. Roommates have noted that slight noises may trigger an episode. His review of systems and past medical history were unremarkable.

Questions

What Is the Differential Diagnosis?
Many conditions can present with complex behaviors arising from the sleep period. These include disorders of arousal (confusional arousals, sleepwalking, or sleep terrors), REM sleep behavior disorder, nocturnal seizures, and psychogenic dissociative disorders [22].

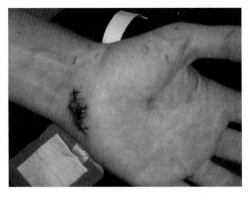

Fig. 2. Disorder of arousal injury. This is a photograph of the injury sustained by this patient when he thrust his hand through a window during a sleepwalking episode.

Disorders of arousal are the most impressive and most frequent of the parasomnias. These share common features: they tend to arise from slow-wave sleep (stages 3 and 4 of NREM sleep), therefore usually occurring in the first third of the sleep cycle (and rarely during naps), and they are common in childhood, usually decreasing in frequency with increasing age. There is often a family history of disorders of arousal; however, this association has recently been questioned. Although they most frequently occur during stages 3 and 4 of NREM sleep (slow-wave sleep), disorders of arousal may occur during any stage of NREM sleep and may occur late in the sleep period [23]. Disorders of arousal occur on a broad spectrum ranging from confusional arousals, to somnambulism (sleepwalking), to sleep terrors. Some take the form of "specialized" behaviors, such as sleep-related eating and sleep-related sexual activity, without conscious awareness [24,25].

Persistence of these behaviors beyond childhood or their development in adulthood is often taken as an indication of significant psychopathology [26,27]. Numerous studies have dispelled this myth, indicating that significant psychopathology is usually not present in adults with disorders of arousal [28–30].

Although usually benign, these behaviors may be violent, resulting in considerable injury to the victim or others or damage to the environment, occasionally with forensic implications [31].

What Studies Should Be Done?

Given the high prevalence of these disorders in normal individuals, formal sleep center evaluation should be confined to those cases in which the behaviors are potentially injurious or violent, extremely bothersome to other household members, result in symptoms of EDS, or have unusual clinical characteristics. In general, if the behaviors are bothersome enough to warrant treatment, then formal sleep studies are indicated to establish a specific diagnosis. Formal sleep studies should include a full EEG seizure montage, with interpretation by an appropriately trained and experienced sleep medicine clinician.

Should This Be Treated? If So, How?

Treating disorders of arousal is often not necessary. Reassurance of their typically benign nature, lack of psychological significance, and the tendency to diminish over time is often sufficient. Tricyclic antidepressants and benzodiazepines may be effective and should be administered if the behaviors are dangerous to person or property or extremely disruptive to family members. Paroxetine and trazodone have been reported effective in isolated cases of disorders of arousal. Nonpharmacologic treatment such as psychotherapy, progressive relaxation, or hypnosis is recommended for long-term management. Anticipatory awakening has been reported to be effective in treating sleepwalking in children. The avoidance of precipitants such as drugs, alcohol, and sleep deprivation is also important [23].

Case 5: REM Sleep Behavior Disorder

A 54-year-old man was seen in the sleep clinic at the urging of his wife. For the past 1.5 years he has experienced progressively worsening dream-enacting behaviors. He reported vivid dreams, which he acts out, resulting in thrashing, punching, and kicking injurious to his wife. The content of the dreams usually involved some type of defensive behavior where he feels that his farm is being invaded by animals or by other human beings. His only medication was lisinopril for mild hypertension. A detailed neurologic evaluation was completely normal. Specifically, there was no evidence of extrapyramidal dysfunction.

Questions

What Is the Differential Diagnosis?

Numerous conditions may result in complex or potentially violent/injurious behaviors arising from the sleep period. These include disorders of arousal (confusional arousals, sleepwalking, or sleep terrors), REM sleep behavior disorder (RBD), nocturnal seizures, sleep apnea, psychogenic dissociative disorders, or malingering. This patient's history of injurious dream-enacting behavior is highly suggestive of RBD.

RBD is a fascinating experiment in nature predicted by animal experiments in 1965.

The typical complaint of a patient with RBD is violent dream-enacting behaviors that are potentially injurious to the individual or bed partner. There are acute and chronic forms of RBD. Acute RBD is almost always induced by medications (tricyclic antidepressants, monoamine oxidase inhibitors, SSRIs, or venlafaxine) or associated with their withdrawal (alcohol, barbiturate, or meprobamate).

RBD most frequently presents with the complaint of dramatic, violent, potentially injurious motor activity during sleep. These behaviors include talking, yelling, swearing, grabbing, punching, kicking, jumping, or running out of the bed. Injuries are not uncommon and include ecchymoses, lacerations, or fractures involving the individual or bed partner. The violence of the sleep-related behavior is often discordant with the waking personality. The reported motor activity usually correlates with remembered dream mentation, leading to the complaint of "acting out my dreams." Less frequently, the primary complaint is one of sleep interruption. The duration of behaviors is brief, and upon awakening from an episode there is usually rapid return of alertness and orientation. Some patients adopt extraordinary measures to prevent injury during sleep: they may tether themselves to the bed with a rope or belt, sleep in sleeping bags, or sleep on a mattress on the floor in a room without furniture. The older (above age 50) and male predominance (80% to 90%) in RBD is overwhelming, although women and virtually all age groups are represented.

Systematic study of patients with neurologic syndromes indicates that RBD and REM sleep without atonia may be far more prevalent than previously suspected. The chronic form of RBD is idiopathic in less than half of occurrences. The remainder are associated with various neurologic disorders, most notably the synucleinopathies (Parkinson's disease, multiple system atrophy, including olivopontocerebellar degeneration and the Shy-Drager syndrome, and dementia with Lewy body disease). RBD may precede the appearance of other symptoms of these disorders by a decade or more [32].

What Studies Should Be Done?

Formal PSG evaluation with a full seizure montage is indicated. This patient's PSG revealed no sleep apnea and no electrical or clinical seizure activity. Prominent tonic and phasic EMG activity was present in both arms and legs during REM sleep, associated with frequent twitching movements and vocalization (Fig. 3). This observation of REM sleep without atonia coupled with the clinical history of dream-enacting behavior confirms the diagnosis of RBD.

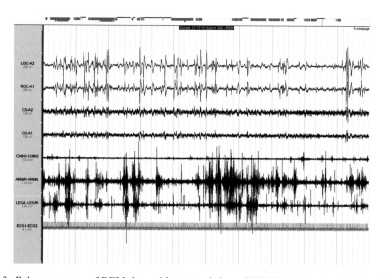

Fig. 3. Polysomnogram of REM sleep without atonia in an REM sleep behavior disorder. Normally during REM sleep there is atonia of all somatic muscles except the diaphragm. This PSG sample shows prominent tonic and phasic EMG activity of the arms and legs during REM sleep (REM sleep without atonia) in a patient with REM sleep behavior disorder. LOC/ROC, left, right outer canthus; A1, A2, left, right ear; C3, left central EEG; O2, right occipital EEG; chin, submental EMG; arms, left, right extensor digitorum EMG; legs, left, right anterior tibialis EMG; ECG, electrocardiogram.

How Should This Be Treated?

The acute form of RBD is self-limited following discontinuation of the offending medication or completion of withdrawal. About 90% of patients with chronic RBD respond well to clonazepam administered one-half hour before sleep time. The dose ranges from 0.5 to 2.0 mg, and there has been little, if any, tendency to develop tolerance, dependence, abuse, or adverse sleep effects despite years of continuous administration and efficacy. Melatonin has also been reportedly effective [32]. Due to the large percentage of patients with RBD who eventually demonstrate extrapyramidal diseases, annual neurologic evaluation is recommended.

Case 6: Restless Legs Syndrome

A 52-year-old married man was referred to the sleep clinic with the complaint of restless sleep. His complaint began 3 years earlier coincident with his beginning hemodialysis for chronic renal failure. He had difficulty initiating and maintaining sleep. He often got up at night and paced about. Although he denied excessive daytime sleepiness, there was a history of falling asleep driving and during conversations. He also frequently fell asleep while pacing in the middle of the night. On one such occasion, he abruptly was overcome with sleep while standing, fell down to the ground in an awkward position, and fractured several metatarsal bones in his foot. On another, he fell asleep sitting on the edge of his bed; he fell forward, hitting his face on the nightstand and breaking four front teeth. On examination, he was ostensibly severely hypersomnolent, having difficulty maintaining enough alertness to participate in the clinical interview.

There was no clinical history to suggest either sleep apnea or narcolepsy. A review of his family medical history revealed that his father and brother both had restless legs syndrome. Initially, the patient received empiric treatment for insomnia, including prescriptions for clonazepam, triazolam, zolpidem, and sertraline. These attempts at treatment for presumptive insomnia were all without any benefit. He had undergone a formal sleep study elsewhere, but no diagnosis or management strategy was offered, as only 11 minutes of sleep occurred during the study.

His sleep was so disrupted that it severely interfered with his wife's sleep—to the extent that she became chronically sleep-deprived, once falling asleep while driving, crashed her car and sustaining severe injuries that resulted in a spinal cord transection with permanent paraplegia.

Questions

What Is the Differential Diagnosis?

Few causes of insomnia result in such severe hypersomnia. Two possibilities come to mind: obstructive sleep apnea and severe restless legs syndrome with periodic extremity movements during sleep. Either or both of these are highly likely in this patient, as these conditions are extremely prevalent in patients with chronic renal failure on dialysis [33].

What Studies Should Be Done?

Formal sleep studies are clearly indicated in view of the dire consequences of the patient's sleepiness. A 3-week actigraphic study revealed no identifiable sleep periods.

The first PSG was difficult to interpret because of the patient's nearly complete inability to initiate or maintain sleep due to periodic movements involving the entire body (Fig. 4). The total sleep time was 285 minutes with a sleep efficiency of 48%. During periods of apparent wakefulness he was obviously confused and disoriented. While sitting on the edge of the bed, he frequently fell asleep, falling backward into bed, hitting the side rails. In retrospect, the lack of apparent sleep on the actigraphic study was due to the prominent periodic extremity movements, which were severe enough to involve the entire body. A second PSG study the next night was nearly identical. During the day, following these studies, he was profoundly hypersomnolent, virtually unable to maintain wakefulness even during stimulation. Because he could not care for himself in this state, he was admitted to the hospital for observation and further study.

Before a third PSG the next night, he was given oxycodone and pramipexole, with marked improvement in sleep continuity. He was discharged

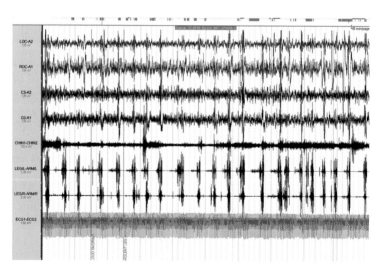

Fig. 4. Polysomngram of severe periodic leg movement in patient with restless legs syndrome. This is a polysomnographic sample of prominent periodic movements of sleep demonstrating severe sleep fragmentation associated with periodic movements involving the entire body. LOC/ROC, left, right outer canthus; A1, A2, left, right ear; C3, left central EEG; O2, right occipital EEG; chin, submental EMG; arms, left, right extensor digitorum EMG; legs, left, right anterior tibialis EMG; ECG, electrocardiogram.

from the hospital on oxycodone and pramipexole with nearly complete resolution of the insomnia and EDS.

What Is the Diagnosis?

This represents an extreme case of restless legs syndrome (RLS). RLS is a neurologic sensory/movement disorder that presents as severe insomnia. RLS is characterized primarily by a vague and difficult-to-describe unpleasant sensation involving the lower extremities. This discomfort appears primarily during periods of inactivity, particularly during the transition from wake to sleep. Patients often have difficulty describing the unpleasant sensations; they rarely use conventional terms of discomfort, such as "numbness, tingling, or pain," but rather bizarre terms such as "pulling, searing, drawing, crawling, or boring," suggesting that the sensations are unlike any experienced by unaffected individuals. These distressing sensations are typically relieved only by movement or stimulation of the legs. Many coping techniques have been found by patients: walking or stomping the feet; rubbing, squeezing, or stroking the legs; taking hot showers or baths; or applying ointment, hot packs, or wraps to the legs. Although these maneuvers are effective while they are being performed, the discomfort usually returns as soon as the individual becomes inactive or returns to bed. The symptoms may also involve the trunk or upper extremities, but usually to a lesser degree than the legs. Those more severely affected may find it extremely difficult to sit for prolonged periods of time, such as during long performances, car trips, or plane rides. The motor restlessness often appears to follow a circadian pattern, peaking between midnight and 4 am [34].

RLS is common, affecting between 5% and 15% of the general population. It may begin in childhood, but tends to be more prevalent with increasing age. It affects men and women. Its association with menstruation, pregnancy, and menopause may explain the female predominance. The prevalence appears to increase with age, but retrospective analysis indicates that symptom onset may begin before the age of 20 in 43% [35,36].

Most cases of RLS are idiopathic or familial. A positive family history may be obtained in up to 50% of cases. Hormonal influences are suggested by the history of exacerbation during menstruation, pregnancy, or menopause. Up to 27% of pregnant women may experience RLS. Although RLS has been associated with a wide variety of other medical and neurologic conditions, such as iron deficiency anemia and various peripheral neuropathies, such cases appear to be uncommon. RLS associated with iron deficiency has been reported following multiple blood donations [37]. RLS affects 20% to 40% of patients with chronic renal failure on dialysis, and may be extraordinarily bothersome, to the extent of interfering with dialysis treatments [38,39]. The RLS symptoms disappear following successful renal transplantation [40]. Extensive and expensive medical and neurologic evaluations are not warranted unless there are historic or physical examination suggestions of other medical disorders. Hemoglobin, serum iron, iron saturation, and ferritin determinations should be obtained to look for mild degrees of anemia [41,42]. Low ferritin levels may be associated with either the development or exacerbation of RLS. Although once felt to be psychiatric in nature, there is no evidence that RLS is related to any psychological or psychiatric problems.

Evidence is accumulating that some cases of RLS are related to iron metabolism abnormalities within the CNS: some patients have low CSF ferritin levels despite normal serum ferritin levels [43], and MRI-determined brain iron concentrations in the subtantia nigra and putamen are reduced [44].

RLS is often confused with periodic limb movements of sleep (PLMS). RLS is a clinical symptom often resulting in severe insomnia, whereas PLMS is a polysomnographic observation, which may or may not have clinical significance. The reason for the confusion that most patients (80%) with RLS have the polysomnographic finding of PLMS; however, the converse is not true [34].

RLS is one of the most important causes of insomnia because of its prevalence and its response to treatment. Most cases of RLS respond gratifyingly to medical treatment, and there are four main classes of medications that are effective [45]:

Anti-Parkinson medications, such as L-Dopa/carbidopa, bromocriptine, pergolide, pramipexole, ropinirole, cabergoline, or selegiline
Benzodiazepines, such as diazepam, clonazepam, temazepam, or triazolam
Opiates, such as codeine, oxycodone, methadone, tramadol, or propoxyphene
Anticonvulsants, such as carbamazepine, gabapentin, or lamotrigine
Intravenous iron

Specific treatment for iron-deficiency anemia is indicated if present.

How Should This Be Managed?
In view of the objective improvement in the patient's sleep while receiving oxycodone and pramipexole, these medications were continued, with nearly immediate and complete resolution of his insomnia and profound sleepiness.

Case 7: Delayed Sleep-Phase Syndrome

A 29-year-old woman was referred to the sleep clinic to evaluate the complaint of an inability to fall asleep at a conventional time and severe difficulty awakening in the morning. She recalled that even as a child she often could not fall asleep until 1 am to 5 am and would be unable to awaken at a "reasonable" time in the morning. She recently lost her job as a teaching assistant as a result of her inability to awaken early enough to get to work on time, despite using multiple alarm clocks and arranging to receive numerous telephone calls in the morning to attempt to awaken her. She was currently working an evening shift between 4 pm and 10 pm without difficulty. With this work schedule, she went to sleep between 2 am and 4 am and slept without interruption until noon or 2 pm. She has a history of depression and bipolar affective disorder, under adequate control at the time of examination.

Questions

What Is the Diagnosis?

The most likely diagnosis is delayed sleep-phase syndrome (DSPS). This is the most common of the circadian rhythm disorders seen in sleep medicine clinics, typically presenting as either sleep-onset insomnia or excessive daytime sleepiness (especially in the morning). The patients with DSPS will often state that if they are allowed to sleep at their preferred time, there are no wake-sleep complaints. It is the timing, not the quality or quantity of sleep, that is problematic. Onset is often during adolescence, but some patients report onset in childhood. A history of DSPS in family members has been noted clinically. The differential diagnosis includes irregular sleep wake pattern and psychiatric disorders associated with disturbed sleep, such as major depression, mania, dysthymia, obsessive-compulsive disorder, and schizophrenia, as well as obstructive sleep apnea syndrome, narcolepsy (particularly during its development in adolescents), and the periodic limb movement disorder with or without the restless legs syndrome [46].

What Studies Should Be Done?

An actigraphic study performed when the patient is allowed to sleep without time constraints usually confirms the diagnosis (Fig. 5). Actigraphic documentation may be valuable in convincing employers or school officials of the organic nature of this condition, so the patient's schedule may be altered to accommodate the biological clock.

How Should This Be Treated?

The administration of melatonin 5 to 7 hours before desired sleep onset and bright light exposure upon awakening have been shown to be effective in advancing sleep onset [47,48]. If melatonin is to be effective in advancing the sleep phase in DSPS, a dose range of 0.3 to 3.0 appears to be adequate.

Case 8: Nocturnal Seizures

A 39-year-old man with mild developmental delay was brought by his parents to the sleep clinic for evaluation of a 10-year history of unusual behaviors during his sleep, typically occurring approximately once monthly, but occasionally on subsequent nights. Within 15 to 20 minutes of going to bed, he begins moaning. His parents find him wandering about his bedroom confused and agitated, with frothy sputum around his mouth. He then develops stereotypic movements of scratching and reaching for things that

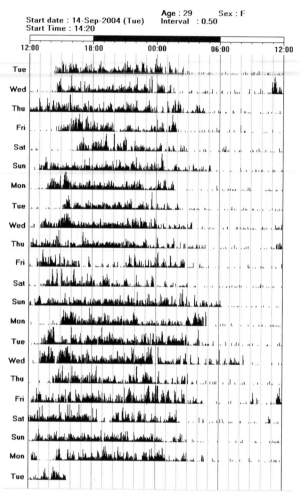

Fig. 5. Actigraphic study of delayed sleep phase syndrome. This is an actigraphic study of a patient with a severe delayed sleep phase syndrome showing late sleep onsets, typically between 3 am and 6 am, with resultant delayed sleep offsets, typically between noon and 3 pm.

are not there. Often he falls during these episodes, and his parents worry about his falling down the stairs leading from his bedroom. Following these episodes, he gradually becomes fully awake after 30 minutes. Because of the potential for injury, his parents had been unwilling to leave him alone at home. They were unable to travel to the family cabin.

There was no history of seizures. He was gainfully employed as a janitor. He underwent a sleep study elsewhere and was found to have mild obstructive sleep apnea. He was placed on nasal CPAP with no improvement in these spells.

Questions

What Is the Differential Diagnosis?

Numerous conditions can result in complex behaviors arising during the sleep period. These include disorders of arousal (confusional arousals, sleepwalking, sleep terrors), REM sleep behavior disorder, obstructive sleep apnea, nocturnal seizures, psychogenic dissociative disorders, or malingering [22].

What Studies Should Be Done?

Because it may be impossible on clinical grounds to differentiate among the various parasomnias, formal sleep studies with a full EEG seizure montage are mandatory, with interpretation by an appropriately trained and experienced sleep medicine clinician.

This patient's formal PSG with full seizure montage was unremarkable. No abnormal behaviors occurred during the study. No EEG abnormalities were present, and normal atonia was present during REM sleep.

What Is the Diagnosis?

Because sleep and epilepsy are closely related, it stands to reason that sleep disorders may mimic, cause, or even be triggered by epileptic phenomena, and vice versa. It is known that, in some individuals, sleep potentiates seizures, as does sleep deprivation [49,50]. In most cases, epilepsy is highly state-dependent: non–rapid-eye-movement (NREM) sleep promotes seizures, whereas rapid-eye-movement (REM) sleep is an antiepileptic state [51,52]. This reflects the dramatic reorganization of the entire central nervous system as it moves across the three states of being: wakefulness, NREM sleep, and REM sleep.

Nocturnal frontal lobe epilepsy (NFLE) may be particularly difficult to diagnose. NFLE, sometimes autosomal dominant, presents a broad spectrum of behaviors, including frequent isolated paroxysmal arousals, episodic nocturnal wanderings, and nocturnal paroxysmal dystonia [53–56]. Temporal lobe seizures may also result in hyperkinetic behaviors [57]. The disorders of arousal may difficult to differentiate from nocturnal seizures, and vice versa [58,59].

In this case, the formal sleep study did not identify a specific diagnosis. Given the recurrent, stereotyped, and inappropriate nature of his sleep-related behaviors, nocturnal seizures were felt to be a likely possibility.

How Should This Be Managed?

Because of the high likelihood that these spells represented nocturnal seizures, the patient was placed on carbamazepine 200 mg at HS with immediate and sustained complete cessation of these spells. His parents can now leave him home alone so they can enjoy their cabin. Patients with exclusively nocturnal seizures may only require antiepileptic medication immediately before bedtime.

Case 9: Sleep-Related Eating Disorder

A 30-year-old happily married woman with inconsequential sleepwalking during childhood and early adolescence presents with a 3-year history of episodes of eating arising from the sleep period, associated with partial amnesia. During these events, she ate peanut butter, cheese, crackers, chips, pasta, chocolate, and ice cream, but virtually never vegetables or fruit. (In contrast, during the day she had always eaten in a healthful manner and had maintained a trim figure). At first she had sporadic sleep-related eating episodes (one to three times weekly), but eventually she was eating once or twice nightly. She attributed a 12-pound weight gain over the past year to her nocturnal eating. She denied feelings of hunger preceding the eating episodes. There was no history suggestive of restless legs syndrome. She did not snore and denied excessive daytime sleepiness. She kept a high level of functioning with a busy life. Her family history was negative for sleep or eating disorders. Her past medical history was normal. There was no history of a diurnal eating disorder.

She slept in the same bed as her husband who reported no other sleep problem. She was a still and quiet sleeper apart from the one to two nightly eating episodes.

Questions

What Is the Differential Diagnosis?

This most likely represents a case of sleep-related eating disorder (SRED). This condition is seen most frequently in women and is usually not associated with an underlying primary eating disorder or with major psychiatric conditions. It may best be thought of as a specialized form of sleepwalking. The eating episodes are associated with varying degrees of awareness. SRED may also be the manifestation of another sleep disorder, such as sleep apnea or restless legs syndrome [24]. Zolpidem has been implicated in triggering SRED [60].

What Studies Should Be Done?

In view of the association between SRED and other sleep disorders, formal PSG studies are recommended to rule out sleep apnea or restless legs syndrome with or without periodic extremity movements of sleep. This patient declined PSG study.

What Is the Treatment?

SRED may respond to a combination of a dopaminergic agent and an opiate or a topiramate [61]. This patient responded well to topiramate.

References

[1] Mitler MM, Carskadon MA, Hirshkowitz M. Evaluating sleepiness. In: Kryger MH, Roth T, Dement WC, editors. Principles and practice of sleep medicine. 4th edition. Philadelphia: Elsevier Saunders; 2005. p. 1417–23.

[2] Aldrich MS. The neurobiology of narcolepsy. Prog Neurobiol 1992;41:538–41.

[3] Taheri S, Zeitzer JM, Mignot E. The role of hypocretins (orexins) in sleep regulation and narcolepsy. Annu Rev Neurosci 2002;25:283–313.

[4] Mignot E, Lammers GJ, Ripley B, Okun M, Nevsimalova S, Overeem S, et al. The role of cerebrospinal fluid hypocretin measurement in the diagnosis of narcolepsy and other hypersomnias. Arch Neurol 2002;59:1553–62.

[5] Nobili L, Ferrillo F, Besset A, Rosadini G, Schiavi G, Billiard M. Ultradian aspects of sleep in narcolepsy. Neurophysiol Clin 1996;26:51–9.

[6] Nishino S, Mignot E. Pharmacological aspects of human and canine narcolepsy. Prog Neurobiol 1997;52:27–78.

[7] American Sleep Disorders Association. Practice parameters for the use of stimulants in the treatment of narcolepsy. Sleep 1994;17:348–51.

[8] Goldman LS, Genel M, Bexman RJ, Slanetz PJ. Diagnosis and treatment of attention-deficit/hyperactivity disorder in children and adolescents. JAMA 1998;279:1100–7.

[9] Pawluk LK, Hurwitz TD, Schluter JL, Ullevig C, Mahowald MW. Psychiatric morbidity in narcoleptics on chronic high dose methylphenidate therapy. J Nerv Ment Dis 1995;183:45–8.

[10] Wallin MT, Mahowald MW. Blood pressure effects of long-term stimulant use in disorders of hypersomnolence. J Sleep Res 1998;7:209–15.

[11] US Xyrem Multicenter Study Group. A randomized, double blind, placebo-controlled multicenter trial comparing the effects of three doses of orally administered sodium oxybate with placebo for the treatment of narcolepsy. Sleep 2002;25:42–9.

[12] US Xyrem Multicenter Study Group. A 12-month, open-label, multicenter extension trial of orally administered sodium oxybate for the treatment of narcolepsy. Sleep 2003;26:31–5.

[13] Thirumalai SS, Shubin RA. The use of citalopram in resistant cataplexy. Sleep Med 2000;1: 313–6.

[14] Salin-Pascual RJ. Improvement in cataplexy and daytime somnolence in narcoleptic patients with venlafaxine XR administration. Sleep and Hypnosis 2002;4:22–5.

[15] Bassetti C, Pelayo R, Guillemiault C. Idiopathic hypersomnia. In: Kryger MH, Roth T, Dement WC, editors. Principles and practice of sleep medicine. 4th edition. Philadelphia: Elsevier Saunders; 2005. p. 791–800.

[16] Janjua T, Samp T, Cramer-Bornemann M, Hannon H, Mahowald MW. Clinical caveat: prior sleep deprivation can affect the MSLT for days. Sleep Med 2003;4:69–72.

[17] Ohayon MM, Roth T. Place of insomnia in the course of depressive and anxiety disorders. J Psychiatr Res 2003;37:9–15.

[18] Bonnet MH, Arand DL. Activity, arousal, and the MSLT in patients with insomnia. Sleep 2000;23:205–12.

[19] Stepanski E, Zorick F, Roehrs T, Young D, Roth T. Daytime alertness in patients with chronic insomnia compared with asymptomatic control subjects. Sleep 1998;11:54–60.

[20] American Academy of Sleep Medicine. International classification of sleep disorders: diagnostic and coding manual. 2nd edition. Westchester (IL): American Academy of Sleep Medicine; 2005.

[21] Ancoli-Israel S. Actigraphy. In: Kryger MH, Roth T, Dement WC, editors. Principles and practice of sleep medicine. 4th edition. Philadelphia: Elsevier Saunders; 2005. p. 1459–67.

[22] Mahowald MW, Cramer Bornemann M, Schenck CH. Parasomnias. Semin Neurol 2004;24: 283–92.

[23] Mahowald MW, Schenck CH. NREM sleep parasomnias. Neurol Clin 2005;23:1077–106.

[24] Schenck CH, Mahowald MW. Review of nocturnal sleep-related eating disorders. Int J Eat Disord 1994;15:343–56.

[25] Shapiro CM, Trajanovic NN, Fedoroff JP. Sexsomnia—a new parasomnia? Can J Psychiatry 2003;48:311–7.

[26] Kales JD, Kales A, Soldatos CR. Night terrors. Clinical characteristics and personality factors. Arch Gen Psychiatry 1980;47:1413–7.

[27] Soldatos CR, Kales A. Sleep disorders: research in psychopathology and its practical implications. Acta Psychiatr Scand 1982;65:381–7.

[28] Schenck CH, Hurwitz TD, Bundlie SR, Mahowald MW. Sleep-related injury in 100 adult patients: a polysomnographic and clinical report. Am J Psychiatry 1989;146:1166–73.

[29] Guilleminault C, Moscovitch A, Leger D. Forensic sleep medicine: nocturnal wandering and violence. Sleep 1995;18:740–8.

[30] Llorente MD, Currier MB, Norman S, Mellman TA. Night terrors in adults: phenomenology and relationship to psychopathology. J Clin Psychiatry 1992;53:392–4.

[31] Mahowald MW, Schenck CH. Violent parasomnias: forensic medicine issues. In: Kryger MH, Roth T, Dement WC, editors. Principles and practice of sleep medicine. 4th edition. Philadelphia: Elsevier Saunders; 2005. p. 960–8.

[32] Schenck CH, Mahowald MW. REM sleep parasomnias. Neurol Clin 2005;23:1107–26.

[33] Parker KP. Sleep disturbances in dialysis patients. Sleep Med Rev 2003;7:131–43.

[34] Montplaisir J, Allen RP, Walters AS, Ferini-Strambi L. Restless legs syndrome and periodic limb movements during sleep. In: Kryger MH, Roth T, Dement WC, editors. Principles and practice of sleep medicine. 4th edition. Philadelphia: Elsevier Saunders; 2005. p. 839–52.

[35] Montplaisir J, Boucher S, Poirier G, Lavigne G, Lapierre O, Lesperance P. Clinical, polysomnographic, and genetic characteristics of restless legs syndrome: a study of 133 patients diagnosed with new standard criteria. Mov Disord 1997;12:61–5.

[36] Phillips B, Young T, Finn L, Asher K, Hening WA, Purvis C. Epidemiology of restless legs symptoms in adults. Arch Intern Med 2000;160(14):2137–41.

[37] Silber MH, Richardson JW. Multiple blood donations associated with iron deficiency in patients with restless legs syndrome. Mayo Clin Proc 2003;78:52–4.

[38] Sandyk R, Bernick C, Lee SM, Stern LZ, Iacono RP, Bamford CR. L-dopa in uremic patients with the restless legs syndrome. Int J Neurosci 1987;35:233–5.

[39] Wetter TC, Stiasny K, Kohnen R, Oertel WH, Trenkwalder C. Polysomnographic sleep measures in patients with uremic and idiopathic restless legs syndrome. Mov Disord 1998; 13:820–4.

[40] Winkelmann J, Stautner A, Samtleben W, Trenkwalder C. Long-term course of restless legs syndrome in dialysis patients after kidney transplantation. Mov Disord 2002;17:1072–6.

[41] Sun ER, Chen CA, Ho G, Earley CJ, Allen RP. Iron and the restless legs syndrome. Sleep 1998;21:371–7.

[42] Aul EA, Davis BJ, Rodnitzky RL. The importance of formal serum iron studies in the assessment of restless legs syndrome. Neurology 1998;51:912.

[43] Earley CJ, Connor JR, Beard JL, Malecki EA, Epstein DK, Allen RP. Abnormalities in CSF concentrations of ferritin and transferritin in restless legs syndrome. Neurology 2000;54: 1698–700.

[44] Allen RP, Barker PB, Wehrl F, Song HK, Earley CJ. MRI measurement of brain iron in patients with restless legs syndrome. Neurology 2001;56:263–5.

[45] Silber MH. Restless legs syndrome. Mayo Clin Proc 1999;72:261–4.

[46] Mahowald MW, Ettinger MG. Circadian rhythm disorders. In: Chokroverty S, editor. Sleep disorders medicine. 3rd edition. Boston: Butterworth Heinemann, in press.

[47] Mundey K, Benloucif S, Harsanyi K, Dubocovich ML, Zee PC. Phase-dependent treatment of delayed sleep phase syndrome with melatonin. Sleep 2005;28:1271–8.

[48] Revell VL, Burgess HJ, Gazda CJ, et al. Advancing human circadian rhythms with afternoon melatonin and morning intermittent bright light. J Endocrinol Metab 2006;91: 54–9.

[49] Dinner D. Effect of sleep on epilepsy. J Clin Neurophysiol 2002;19:504–13.

[50] Mendez M, Radtke RA. Interactions between sleep and epilepsy. J Clin Neurophysiol 2001; 18:106–27.

[51] Shouse MN, Siegel JM, Wu FM, Szymusiak R, Morrison AR. Mechanisms of seizure suppression during rapid-eye-movement (REM) sleep in cats. Brain Res 1989;505:271–82.

[52] Shouse MN, da Silva AM, Sammaritano M. Circadian rhythm, sleep, and epilepsy. J Clin Neurophysiol 1996;13:32–50.

[53] Provini F, Plazzi G, Tinuper P, Vandi S, Lugaresi E, Montagna P. Nocturnal frontal lobe epilepsy: a clinical and polygraphic overview of 100 consecutive cases. Brain 1999; 122(Pt 6):1017–31.

[54] Provini F, Plazzi G, Montagna P, Lugarelsi E. The wide clinical spectrum of nocturnal frontal lobe epilepsy. Sleep Med Rev 2000;4:375–86.

[55] Oldani A, Zucconi M, Asselta R, Modugno M, Bonati MT, Dalpra L, et al. Autosomal dominant nocturnal frontal lobe epilepsy. A video-polysomnographic and genetic appraisal of 40 patients and delineation of the epileptic syndrome. Brain 1998;121:205–23.

[56] Scheffer IE, Bhatia KP, Lopes-Cendes I, Fish DR, Marsden CD, Andermann E, et al. Autosomal dominant nocturnal frontal lobe epilepsy. A distinctive clinical disorder. Brain 1995; 118(Pt 1):61–73.

[57] Nobili L, Cossu M, Mai R, Tassi L, Cardinale F, Castana L, et al. Sleep-related hyperkinetic seizures of temporal lobe origin. Neurology 2004;62:482–5.

[58] Pedley TA. Differential diagnosis of episodic symptoms. Epilepsia 1983;24(Suppl 1):S31–44.

[59] Lombroso CT. Pavor nocturnus of proven epileptic origin. Epilepsia 2000;41:1221–6.

[60] Schenck CH, Connoy DA, Castellanos M, Johnson B, Werner R, Wills L, et al. Zolpidem-induced amnestic sleep-related eating disorder (SRED) in 19 patients [abstract]. Sleep 2005; 28:A259.

[61] Winkelman JW. Treatment of nocturnal eating syndrome and sleep-related eating disorder with topiramate. Sleep Med 2003;4:243–6.

ELSEVIER
SAUNDERS

Neurol Clin 24 (2006) 291–307

NEUROLOGIC
CLINICS

Epilepsy Case Studies

Edward Faught, MD[a,b,]*

[a]*Department of Neurology, University of Alabama School of Medicine,
Birmingham, AL, USA*
[b]*University of Alabama at Birmingham Epilepsy Center, Birmingham, AL, USA*

Seizures are the second most common neurologic condition, after headache. All physicians encounter patients who have seizures and may be called on to treat them. Therefore, a basic knowledge of seizure types, causes, and treatment strategies is useful. It also is helpful to be able to recognize some of the common epilepsy syndromes. This article reviews the definitions and terminology of seizures and epilepsy syndromes and uses case histories to describe typical scenarios likely to be encountered by primary care physicians and neurologists.

Definitions

A *seizure* is a brief disturbance of cerebral function, lasting from seconds to a few minutes, caused by an abnormal electrical discharge. *Epilepsy* is the tendency to have seizures on a chronic, recurrent basis, not resulting from a temporary condition. The term, epilepsy, does not presuppose a cause; there are myriad causes. Essentially, anything that disturbs the normal functioning of the cerebral cortex can cause seizures, and if this abnormality is enduring, it can result in epilepsy. Epilepsy affects approximately 1% of children and 0.5% of adults [1]. The difference results primarily from the

The author has received research support, honoraria for speaking, and consulting fees from Abbott Laboratories, GlaxoSmithKline, Johnson and Johnson, Novartis, Ortho McNeil, and Pfizer. He has received honoraria for speaking and consulting fees from Shire and UCB Pharma. He has received research support from Eisai, Schwarz, the National Institutes of Health, and the Department of Veterans Affairs. No financial support was received for the preparation of this manuscript, but the companies listed manufacture products described in the text, and the companies and institutions listed have sponsored research studies referenced in the text.

* UAB Epilepsy Center, Civitan International Research Center 312, 1719 6th Avenue South, Birmingham, AL 35294-0021, USA.

E-mail address: faught@uab.edu

0733-8619/06/$ - see front matter © 2006 Elsevier Inc. All rights reserved.
doi:10.1016/j.ncl.2006.01.001

fact that some childhood epilepsies remit, although some childhood epilepsy syndromes are fatal.

Seizure types

Seizures are classified into two basic categories, *generalized onset* and *partial onset* (Box 1) [2]. Focal is a synonym for partial in this context. Generalized-onset seizures arise over a wide area of the cortex simultaneously, involve both hemispheres, and, by definition, are associated with immediate loss of consciousness. Partial-onset seizures are those that can be recognized, by clinical or electroencephalographic (EEG) features, to begin in a restricted brain region. A confusing aspect of the terminology is that partial-onset seizures can, and often do, spread to involve the whole cortex and eventuate in a convulsion: a *generalized tonic-clonic seizure*. This event is referred to by the awkward term, secondarily generalized tonic-clonic seizure. Other generalized seizure types are *absence* (a staring spell lasting a few seconds) and *myoclonic* (a brief sudden jerk of the upper body). Less common generalized-onset seizures types are *atonic* (a sudden drop to the ground), *infantile spasms*, and *clonic* or *tonic* seizures.

Partial-onset seizures are either *simple partial*, which involve no change in consciousness, or *complex partial*, which cause a trance-like state lasting 30 to 120 seconds because of involvement of limbic structures subserving awareness and memory. A simple partial seizure can evolve into a complex partial seizure. In this circumstance, the simple partial portion sometimes is referred to as an *aura*.

Box 1. Classification of epileptic seizures

Partial onset
Simple partial (no loss of consciousness)
Complex partial (consciousness altered)
Partial secondarily generalized (culminate in a convulsion)

Generalized onset
Generalized tonic-clonic (a convulsion; grand mal)
Absence (petit mal)
Infantile spasms
Atonic (drop attacks)
Clonic or tonic

Abbreviated from the International Classification of Epileptic Seizures.
Data from Commission on Classification and Terminology of the International League Against Epilepsy. Proposal for revised clinical and electroencephalographic classification of epileptic seizures. Epilepsia 1981;22:489–501.

Laypersons and many physicians refer to generalized tonic-clonic seizures as grand mal seizures. This term no longer is official but is readily understood. The term, petit mal, however, is subject to more confusion. To neurologists, it has the specific meaning of an absence seizure. Patients, however, may refer to any staring spell or minor seizure as a petit mal. It is helpful to remember that absence seizures virtually always arise in early childhood and are seen only in those adults in whom they have persisted since childhood. Seizures causing staring spells in adults almost always are complex partial seizures.

Causes of seizures

Seizures resulting from a transient cause are not referred to as epilepsy. Generalized tonic-clonic seizures are frequent consequences of alcohol or benzodiazepine withdrawal and various metabolic disturbances. Partial-onset seizures occurring immediately or in the first few days after head trauma or stroke often subside spontaneously and do not result in epilepsy.

Generalized-onset seizures often are caused by genetic syndromes and often, but not always, manifest first during childhood. Partial-onset seizures can arise at any age and most often are caused by an acquired brain lesion (trauma, infection, tumor, stroke, and so forth). In recent years, however, a few epilepsy syndromes characterized by partial-onset seizures have been recognized as inherited [3]. A cause for epilepsy can be determined or reasonably suspected in only approximately half of cases. This is true for partial and generalized seizure syndromes. This is a source of frustration for patients but does not necessarily preclude effective treatment.

Epilepsy syndromes are recognizable clusters of signs and symptoms with a predictable prognosis and, sometimes, a defined cause [3]. Although epilepsy syndromes include one or more seizure types, this concept goes further, taking into account other patient characteristics. An abbreviated classification of currently recognized epilepsy syndromes is in Box 2.

An illustrative example is childhood absence epilepsy (CAE) [4]. This syndrome often begins at ages 5 to 7. Kindergarten teachers may observe brief lapses of awareness lasting 5 to 20 seconds, after which the child immediately is responsive and alert; these are absence seizures. The seizures often occur multiple times daily and may be mistaken for daydreaming. An EEG reveals a pathognomonic pattern called a three-per-second spike and wave. Treatment with valproic acid (Depakote) or ethosuximide (Zarontin) is highly effective [4], and approximately two thirds of children go into permanent remission before adulthood; they "outgrow" their seizures [5]. Fifty percent of children, however, have occasional generalized tonic-clonic seizures also, and this group is less likely to enter remission [6]. CAE is caused by genetic factors; it probably has a multifactorial genetic cause with age-related expression [7]. There are other epilepsy syndromes, including juvenile absence

---

Box 2. Common epilepsy syndromes

Localization-related (focal, partial; idiopathic, probably genetic)
Benign epilepsy with centrotemporal spikes

Localization related: symptomatic
Temporal lobe epilepsies
   Mesiobasal limbic seizures
   Lateral temporal seizures
Frontal lobe epilepsies
Parietal lobe epilepsies
Occipital lobe epilepsies

Generalized epilepsies (idiopathic, probably genetic)
Childhood absence epilepsy (CAE)
Juvenile absence epilepsy
Benign sylvian-rolandic epilepsy
Juvenile myoclonic epilepsy (JME)
Epilepsy with grand mal seizures on awakening

Generalized epilepsies (cryptogenic or symptomatic)
West syndrome (infantile spasms)
Lennox-Gastaut syndrome

Generalized epilepsies (symptomatic; specific syndromes)
Many disease states complicated by seizure

   Abbreviated from the International Classification of Epilepsies and Epileptic Syndromes.
   Data from Commission on Classification and Terminology of the International League Against Epilepsy. Proposal for classification of epilepsies and epileptic syndromes. Epilepsia 1985;26:268–78.

---

epilepsy (JAE) and juvenile myoclonic epilepsy (JME), which may include absence seizures as one of their manifestations, but they have other features and different prognoses.

Not all patients can be pigeonholed into known epilepsy syndromes. The following cases are designed to illustrate approaches to common clinical situations, some of which are manifestations of specific syndromes and others of which often are encountered but whose cause is less well defined.

Case 1: the first seizure

After an all-night fraternity party at which he drank several beers, a 19-year-old man went to bed at 4:00 AM. His roommate was awakened at 6:00 AM by a commotion and found him "convulsing" in his bed. He "looked blue, foamed at his mouth, and then breathed hard." He was incontinent of urine. An ambulance was called. By the time it arrived, he had awakened but seemed confused. In the emergency department, 1 hour later, he was alert and oriented and, although his muscles were sore, he had no other complaints. Hematology and chemistry tests were normal. A blood alcohol level was low but not zero. A CT scan of his head was normal. A neurologic examination was completely normal.

Questions

Does he have epilepsy?
What other tests should be done?
What is the likelihood that he will have another seizure?
Should he be treated?
What restrictions should be placed on his activity?

Diagnosis of epilepsy

Epilepsy may be defined as a tendency to have seizures on a chronic, recurrent basis. This definition suggests that at least two seizures must occur for a diagnosis of epilepsy and that the seizures are not the result of a transient or temporary condition. According to the first criterion, this young man cannot be said to have epilepsy. Was the convulsion, which sounds by history much like a generalized tonic-clonic seizure, caused by a temporary event or condition? Syncope (fainting) often results in muscle jerking, which usually is brief but can mimic a full-blown convulsion. This is called convulsive syncope. Perhaps this patient was dehydrated from alcohol, but there was no orthostatic change or sudden emotional event to suggest a vasovagal cause for syncope. What was the role of alcohol? Alcohol is well known to lower the seizure threshold, but his blood alcohol level was not especially high. Alcohol withdrawal seizures occur most commonly 12 to 24 hours after the last drink, when the level is zero [8]. There were no other apparent factors except sleep loss. Nevertheless, every person who has epilepsy must have had a first seizure at some point, and the other questions must be addressed.

Evaluation for the cause of a seizure

A search for the cause of the seizure includes blood tests for metabolic problems, such as hypoglycemia, hyponatremia, or hypocalcemia, although these are uncommon in previously healthy people. A urine drug screen should be done, although common drugs of abuse, such as opiates and marijuana, do not cause seizures. Amphetamines and cocaine can produce seizures occasionally. Benzodiazepine withdrawal is a common cause for seizures; recent use should be asked about. Head CT reveals intracranial bleeding and most tumors. Severe headache preceding the seizure may suggest subarachnoid hemorrhage from an aneurysm; CT does not always detect this and a lumbar puncture should be done if this is suspected. Lumbar puncture also is indicated if fever or other signs of meningitis are present. These tests are sufficient for an emergency department evaluation. Two other tests, however—MRI and EEG—should be scheduled as soon as possible. The MRI may reveal an underlying structural cause for the seizure, such as a tumor, abscess, cortical dysplasia, or mesial temporal sclerosis.

Excepting a good eyewitness description, EEG is the only way to make a definite diagnosis of epilepsy. Although recording an actual seizure during a standard 20-minute EEG is unlikely, approximately 50% of people who have epilepsy have an epileptiform EEG abnormality between seizures [9]. The other 50% does not; thus, a normal EEG does not rule out epilepsy.

The major historical feature that should be sought is the occurrence of any previous neurologic insult. This includes head trauma, meningitis, or encephalitis and neurosurgical procedures—occurrences often referred to in the literature as remote symptomatic neurologic events. This history dramatically increases the chance that further seizures will occur, from 17% to 34% in one series [10]. Head trauma, to represent a predisposing event for epilepsy, must be significant. Many people have a history of minor head trauma without loss of consciousness or of mild concussion; these events are not risk factors for epilepsy.

The other important historical distinction is whether or not the seizure was generalized or partial in onset. Partial-onset seizures may have an aura that is recalled by the patient. Depending on the part of the brain involved initially, this may be an unusual sensation, smell, taste, memory, or other "funny feeling." Witnesses may have noticed the onset with an initial stare or jerking starting on one side of the body. Partial-onset seizures suggest an underlying focal structural abnormality of the cortex and are highly likely to recur [10]. Focally abnormal findings after the seizure on neurologic examination have the same significance. An abnormal CT or MRI scan also suggests a fixed lesion, which could be the source for further seizures.

Prognosis after a first seizure

There is an extensive literature on prognosis after a first seizure. The factors increasing the likelihood of recurrence (discussed previously) include abnormal EEG, history of a remote symptomatic neurologic event, and any evidence for a partial (focal) onset. Alternatively, in an otherwise healthy person who has a normal neurologic examination in whom all tests are normal, the chance of having another seizure is low. Among 407 children followed after a first seizure, 42% had another seizure at 5-year follow-up [11]. In another series of 244 patients of all ages, 27% had another seizure within 3 years [10]. In summary, an otherwise healthy person who has a first generalized tonic-clonic seizure has less than a 50% chance of having another one within the next few years.

To treat or not to treat and activity restrictions

Knowledge that a generalized convulsion in a healthy individual stands a good chance of being an isolated, single event should inform the treatment decision. Most neurologists opt for not prescribing medication and adopting a wait-and-see attitude. In most states, however, a driving restriction is mandatory, ranging from 3 to 12 months after a seizure involving loss of consciousness, as in this case. This young man has to be told that he cannot drive for a while, regardless of whether or not medication is prescribed. Other reasonable restrictions include avoidance of heights, working with dangerous machinery, and swimming or bathing alone. Some patients may insist on treatment. If medication is prescribed, however, this simply defers the equally difficult decisions of when to discontinue it and of whether or not restrictions are necessary for some time after treatment is stopped.

Finally, this young man will be concerned, understandably, about what caused the event, even if all tests are negative and he is reassured that recurrence is unlikely. It may help to explain to him that seizures are a nonspecific response of the brain to a variety of stresses and that common stresses are sleep loss and alcohol. It probably also is true that everyone has a certain threshold for having a seizure, on a genetic basis, and that this man may have a lower threshold than average. Consequently, he should be more cautious about late-night partying!

Case 2: a clumsy teenager

A 15-year-old boy, while eating breakfast, suddenly flung his orange juice into the air, cried out loudly, and had a convulsion. He previously was healthy, although his family described him as "clumsy," especially in the mornings. He seemed to drop things often. The initial evaluation, including neurologic examination, blood tests, and MRI scan, was unrevealing. Past history also was unremarkable, although he reported not liking bright lights and feeling "queasy" recently while playing video games.

An EEG was described as abnormal, with a "photoparoxysmal response"— generalized spike-and-wave discharges when a strobe light was turned on at a flash rate of 16 per second. He found the strobe very unpleasant.

Because of the EEG, the family was told that he had a "seizure disorder" and he was given a prescription for carbamazepine (Tegretol). Six weeks later, however, he had another convulsion, and teachers reported that he had begun to "stare into space" during classes.

Questions

Does he have epilepsy?
What type of seizures does he have?
What is his diagnosis?
What caused it?
Why did the carbamazepine not work?

What is the best treatment?
How long does he need to take medication?

Diagnosis

This boy has epilepsy. By definition, he has had at least two seizures not related to a temporary or transient condition. Physicians sometimes use the term, seizure disorder, but this is a euphemism that should be avoided. He and his family need to hear unequivocally that the diagnosis is epilepsy. In the long run, this is in his best interest. It allows the family to access printed and electronic information and to avail themselves of services of the Epilepsy Foundation, which has local chapters in most cities and states.

Seizure types

He has generalized tonic-clonic (grand mal) seizures. The orange-juice flinging and "clumsiness" in this case were further clues: additional questioning led to a description of sudden jerks of the arms, which led to dropping items. These are myoclonic seizures. The staring spells raise the question either of absence seizures (petit mal) or complex partial seizures. The association with the generalized tonic-clonic and myoclonic seizures and the history that the staring spells in school lasted only a few seconds make absence seizures more likely. All of the seizure types in this case are generalized-onset seizures, not partial-onset.

Epilepsy syndrome

An epilepsy syndrome is more than a description of the seizure type or types. It also implies a cause, any associated clinical signs or symptoms, and a prognosis [3]. This patient has a common epilepsy syndrome called JME. JME probably is the most common cause of new-onset seizures among adolescents and, therefore, it is important for primary care physicians and neurologists to be familiar with it [12,13]. This is because it has a specific cause, treatment, and prognosis.

Juvenile myoclonic epilepsy

JME is a genetic disorder, although the specific chromosome and gene involved vary among different pedigrees. Inheritance seems to be complicated, with only 14% of first-degree relatives having the same syndrome [13,14]. A generalized tonic-clonic seizure usually brings patients to a doctor, but a careful history often reveals that myoclonic jerks have been occurring for months or years. These jerks typically are sudden movements of the arms, sometimes the head, and rarely the whole body or legs. They involve elevation and forward flexion of the shoulders and often cause patients to drop or fling objects in the hands. The amplitude varies from small, inapparent movements to huge jerks that can throw a patient to the ground. Absence seizures also occur in approximately 20% of patients who have JME [12,13]. The seizures most often occur early in the morning and are worsened by sleep loss and fatigue. The average age of onset is 14 years, but onsets in early childhood and as late as the 30s are described [12–14]. There is a highly characteristic EEG pattern consisting of bursts of generalized polyphasic spike-and-waves.

JME is the epilepsy syndrome most likely to involve photosensitivity [15]. Patients are typically sensitive to flashing lights of 10 to 20 per second, although this often is demonstrable only in the EEG laboratory [15]. Environmental stimuli, however, also can produce discomfort or actual seizures. The most common real-world stimulus is sunlight flickering through the trees into a moving automobile. Television, video games, and fan blades also may be responsible. Video games do not produce epilepsy, however, in those who are not genetically predisposed to having photosensitive seizures [16].

Treatment

JME usually is easy to treat, responding completely to valproate (Depakote) in 86% of patients [14]. Valproate is effective for all three seizure types. Patients who have side effects from this drug may respond to newer drugs, although none are approved specifically by the Food and Drug Administration (FDA) for this condition. Zonisamide (Zonegran) [17], levetiracetam (Keppra) [18], or topiramate (Topamax) [18] may be effective. Lamotrigine (Lamictal) treats the absence and tonic-clonic seizures [19] but its effect on myoclonus is variable; sometimes it makes it worse [20].

One important reason for classifying seizures accurately is that certain antiepileptic drugs make certain seizure types worse. Carbamazepine (Tegretol or Carbatrol), although a good treatment for generalized tonic-clonic seizures, may worsen myoclonus [21] and absence [22]. This boy's absence attacks were precipitated by the carbamazepine. Other drugs that may do this are gabapentin (Neurontin), tiagabine (Gabatril), and phenytoin (Dilantin) [20].

Treatment of JME must be lifelong. Patients may be lulled into feeling that they can stop their medication after several years of freedom from seizures, but 90% of the time seizures recur [12,13]. It is important, therefore, for physicians to recognize this syndrome and to advise patients accordingly.

Case 3: a young woman who had déjà vu

A 22-year-old woman was referred to an epilepsy center because of intractable seizures. She had had three brief febrile seizures at the age of 2, had taken phenobarbital until age 5, then had no further problems until age 14. She then had a convulsion and was noted to have staring spells. Phenytoin prevented further convulsions, but her acne worsened and she complained of facial hair. She continued to have 2 to 4 staring spells per month; they began with a "rising feeling" in the pit of her stomach, followed by a sudden sense that everything had happened before, then amnesia for the rest of the seizure. At this point, her family described a blank stare, with some lip smacking and aimless pulling at her clothes, for approximately a minute. Afterward she was sleepy and confused for 30 minutes. Eventually, a combination of carbamazepine and valproate reduced the seizure frequency to 2 per month, but maximally tolerated dosages of each drug failed to render her seizure-free. She is engaged and would like to have children.

Questions

What is her seizure type?
In which part of the brain does it likely arise?
Should she have children?
If so, what is an appropriate medical treatment?
Should she consider surgery?

Seizure type

The seizure description is classical for complex partial seizures of temporal lobe origin. In approximately 70% to 80% of patients who have complex partial seizures, the temporal lobe is the culprit; therefore, this syndrome often is referred to as temporal lobe epilepsy [23]. Most temporal lobe seizures originate in the mesial part of one of the lobes, especially the hippocampus. The simple partial onset, if one occurs (the aura) most often is an odd, epigastric rising sensation [23]. Déjà vu, olfactory, or taste phenomena may occur. The lip smacking and clothes picking are examples of automatisms. In particular patients, they tend to be stereotyped, although the repertoire varies considerably between patients. This stereotypy is a clue to the epileptic nature of the events. Patients who have psychogenic episodic behaviors—pseudo-seizures—often manifest different behaviors at different times.

Childbearing with seizures

In the nineteenth century, women (and men) who had epilepsy were sometimes sterilized. This practice continued into the twentieth century in many states [24]. It still is distressingly frequent for women who have epilepsy to be discouraged from having children by their physicians. It now is clear that most such pregnancies produce normal children, but some antiepilepsy medications are teratogens and specific precautions should be taken before pregnancy commences.

Many of the older medications, specifically phenobarbital, carbamazepine, and phenytoin, increase the risk of birth defects by a factor of approximately two [25–27]. There is a 2% to 3% risk of birth defects among children born to women who have epilepsy who are taking no medications; the risk is only slightly higher than in nonepileptic women. Phenobarbital, carbamazepine, and phenytoin raise the rate to 4% to 5% [25–27]. Contrary to previous opinion, there is not a typical anticonvulsant teratogen syndrome; various defects, including cardiac septal defects, facial clefts, and limb anomalies, may occur [25–27]. Valproate should be avoided, if possible, in young women. The Harvard Pregnancy Registry, a prospective registry of women taking antiepilepsy drugs, recently reported a 10.9% rate of birth defects among children of women taking valproate during the first trimester [28]. Newer antiepilepsy drugs may be safer, based on animal studies and limited human experience. The most systematic experience is with lamotrigine; several prospective studies suggest a birth defect rate of approximately 2% to 3%, although the numbers as yet are not statistically significant in comparison to pregnancies in women taking no antiepilepsy drugs [29–31]. At present, the older drugs are FDA category D—known human teratogens, whereas the newer drugs, including lamotrigine, are category C—effects on the fetus unknown. Lamotrigine, however, has the disadvantage that its clearance increases and serum levels drop substantially during pregnancy, requiring frequent serum level testing to avoid increases in seizure frequency [32].

It usually is not a good idea to stop medication when pregnancy is discovered. Generalized tonic-clonic seizures during pregnancy clearly are dangerous for the mother and are associated with increased incidences of pregnancy complications, including miscarriage [25–27]. Nevertheless, it may be possible in some women to withdraw medication cautiously before pregnancy, if no seizures have occurred for several years, and especially if there is no history of convulsions.

Surgery

Surgery is a well-accepted and standard treatment for seizures that do not respond to medication [33,34]. Only surgery for partial-onset seizures potentially is curative, and success depends on precise localization of the seizure focus. This is accomplished by several means, including clinical semiology of the seizures, interictal and ictal EEG recordings, MRI results, and results of other neuroimaging studies [35]. A metanalysis of surgical results reveals a 5-year seizure-free rate of 66% for temporal lobe surgery and 46% for occipital or parietal lobe surgery but only 27% for frontal lobe surgery [36]. The best results are for mesial temporal lobe epilepsy; postoperative seizure-free rates exceeding 70% now are routine at major epilepsy centers [34]. The lesion found most often on pathologic examination is mesial temporal sclerosis. It is unclear what causes this lesion and whether or not it is the cause of the seizures or a result of repeated seizures that have an impact on that area. Mesial temporal sclerosis can be detected with a high degree of accuracy with proper MRI techniques [37].

This patient failed three standard antiepilepsy medications. Should more be tried before surgery? In a recent landmark study, Scottish investigators report that if patients fail to respond to the first two medications because of lack of efficacy (not because of side effects), there is little chance that additional medication trials will render patients seizure-free [37]. Indeed, 36% of patients in this study remained refractory after trials of 3 or more medications, alone or in combination. This means that a large number of patients who have epilepsy do not obtain satisfactory results from medications, and many potentially are good surgical candidates. Surgery for epilepsy is relatively safe [33,34]. This patient should be considered for surgery. It is important for her physicians not to convey the message, overtly or subtly, that surgery is a last resort. It should not take more than 2 or 3 years after diagnosis of epilepsy to establish if a patient is refractory and should be evaluated for surgery, but delays of many years or even decades still are common. This primarily is a problem of physician education.

Not all brain areas are resectable without unacceptable neurologic consequences, and sometimes the seizure focus simply cannot be located with certainty. In those cases, surgery is not an option and continued medication trials are justified. Finally, this patient's best chance at discontinuing medication before planning a pregnancy is to have surgery. Even so, most neurologists continue medications for at least 2 years after surgery, even if no further seizures occur, and some patients recur when they are withdrawn but do well when medication is resumed. For this reason, it still is important to establish the most effective and safest medication regimen even if surgery is contemplated.

Case 4: epilepsy late in life

A 77-year-old right-handed man was brought to his physician because "his mind is wandering," according to his wife. For the previous 2 months, she had noted that he sometimes did not answer for up to a minute when spoken to and sometimes adamantly insisted that he had not heard her say something even though he had looked directly at her when she said it. His history included many years of hypertension with treatment and a small stroke 1 year previously, which left him with only a mild weakness of the left hand. He also had become somewhat "forgetful" during the previous 2 or 3 years, and she had taken over the chore of balancing the checkbook.

On examination, he was alert and oriented but could recall only two of three words 5 minutes later. His hearing was intact. Neurologic examination was normal except for slight weakness and clumsiness of the left hand. An MRI scan of the head revealed small, old cerebral infarctions in the left temporal and right frontal cortical regions and several subcortical white matter hyperintensities. An EEG was normal.

Questions

What is the differential diagnosis of these events?
What other studies should be done?
What is the underlying cause of the events?
How should he be treated?

Differential diagnosis

The history given by this patient's wife does not lead directly to a single diagnosis. Several possibilities come to mind: simple inattention, hearing trouble, daydreaming, some sort of attentional deficit related to a dementing process, transient ischemic attacks (TIAs), or seizures [38]. The first four can be ruled out by asking the wife if she can get his attention during these episodes, if necessary by confronting him face-on and loudly. In this case, she stated that she could not, even by waving her hand in front of his face. After a minute or so, however, he began to answer and make eye contact, although he seemed to be talking and thinking more slowly than usual for up to an hour after each episode.

Could these be TIAs? TIAs, caused by an embolic source or by transient variations in cerebral blood flow, usually last at least several minutes [38]. They may last for hours, although the longer ones increasingly suggest actual cerebral infarction. Carotid circulation TIAs typically produce transient motor weakness (not jerking), sensory change (usually described as numbness, not strange or paresthetic sensations), or monocular blindness. They do not produce changes in awareness because they ordinarily involve only one hemisphere. Vertebrobasilar (posterior circulation) TIAs can alter consciousness if they reduce flow to the rostral brainstem, but usually this is accompanied by other signs or symptoms, such as dizziness, vertigo, diplopia, nausea, or hemifield visual loss. These latter symptoms are uncommon with seizures.

The possibility of seizures in this patient must be considered, specifically, complex partial seizures. Nevertheless, it may seem strange that there is only blank staring, no automatisms, and a normal EEG. To explain this patient's syndrome, some of the characteristics of seizures in the elderly are reviewed. Epilepsy beginning after age 60 differs in several important ways from seizures in the young, and treatment strategies must be modified [39].

Seizures in the elderly

Until a few years ago, it was believed that epilepsy primarily was a disorder of childhood and that the incidence declined progressively throughout life. Careful epidemiologic studies establish that epilepsy is common in the elderly; after age 70, the incidence is higher than in any decade after the first [40,41]. People are living longer, and many survive to develop conditions predisposing to seizures. The major cause of new-onset seizures in the elderly is cerebrovascular disease [41,42].

The most common seizure type in elderly patients is the complex partial seizure [43]. For unknown reasons, automatisms seem to be less prominent than in younger patients who have complex partial seizures [43]. Simple blank staring, therefore, as this patient demonstrates, is not uncommon but presents more of a diagnostic challenge. To add to the problems of diagnosis, the interictal EEG in elderly patients who have epilepsy often is normal [44]. The normal EEG in this patient, therefore, does not rule out epilepsy.

What other tests should be done? Prolonged inpatient EEG recording with simultaneous video, for several days if necessary, is considered the gold standard for diagnosis of epilepsy. It can be useful for diagnosis in elderly patients [45]. That is an option in this case, but sometimes this expensive inpatient test is unavailable locally or is nondiagnostic. In that case, if other reasonable options are ruled out, a therapeutic trial of an antiepilepsy drug may be indicated.

Etiology of epilepsy in the elderly

Cerebrovascular disease is a common cause of seizures in this age group and should be evaluated in any patients developing seizures for the first time after age 60 or in the presence of vascular risk factors. Tests may include carotid and cardiac ultrasounds, electrocardiography, and magnetic resonance angiography of neck and cerebral vessels. In this patient, it is possible that the old temporal stroke could be the source of the complex partial seizures.

Alzheimer's disease is a risk factor for seizures, especially as the dementia advances [46,47], and should be considered in this patient. The normal EEG does not rule that out; EEGs are relatively insensitive to early Alzheimer's. Structural causes, such as neoplasms, aneuryms, and abscesses, can be evaluated by MRI. Metabolic factors should be assessed. However, with the exception of hypoglycemia or hyperglycemia [48], metabolic encephalopathies produce generalized tonic-clonic seizures, not complex partial seizures.

Treatment of seizures in the elderly

The watchword is gentleness. Declines in hepatic and renal function with aging result in greater accumulation and higher serum drug levels for a given dose for many drugs [39,49]. Furthermore, older patients seem to be more subject to central nervous system adverse effects of drugs. This clearly is the case for older drugs, such as phenytoin, phenobarbital, carbamazepine, and valproate [41]. There is a growing belief that newer-generation drugs are tolerated better and, therefore, are more appropriate in the elderly, but many still receive older drugs [50]. Fortunately, seizure control in this population may be achievable with lower drug dosages and lower serum drug concentrations than in most younger patients [39,44,51]. A rule of thumb is to halve the recommended starting dose of antiepilepsy medication for patients over age 60 and to make dose increases at longer intervals. This strategy presumes that there is no urgency to achieve optimal seizure control, which usually is the case with outpatients. Control should not be delayed unduly, but a couple of extra weeks usually are acceptable.

What is the best antiepilepsy drug at this patient's age? Traditional drugs are problematic: the enzyme-inducing drugs, phenytoin, carbamazepine, and phenobarbital, may produce interactions with some of the many other drugs older patients take [52]. Phenytoin may exacerbate gait unsteadiness. Valproate can be used, but it exacerbates essential tremor, if present. A recent large clinical trial sponsored by the United States Department of Veterans Affairs (VA Cooperative Study) addresses this question [53]. A total of 593 patients who had new-onset seizures over the age of 60, mean age 72, were randomized to receive relatively low target dosages of carbamazepine (600 mg), lamotrigine (150 mg), or gabapentin (1500 mg per day) in a blinded multicenter trial. The primary endpoint was satisfactory treatment for 1 year. Although there were no statistically significant differences in seizure control, carbamazepine was less well tolerated: dropouts resulting from adverse drug reactions were 31% for carbamazepine, 22% for gabapentin, and 12% for lamotrigine ($P = 0.001$). Of patients assigned to carbamazepine, 35.5% remained in the study for a year, compared with 49% of those taking gabapentin and 56% of those taking lamotrigine. This difference was statistically significant for carbamazepine versus the other two drugs but not for gabapentin versus lamotrigine. Neither gabapentin nor lamotrigine are FDA approved for initial monotherapy, although lamotrigine is approved for transition to monotherapy. Other newer drugs may be satisfactory but have not been tested rigorously in the elderly. Levetiracetam was well tolerated in small, open-label series [54,55] but is not FDA approved for monotherapy.

References

[1] Tellez-Zenteno JF, Pondal-Sordo M, Metijevic S, et al. National and regional prevalence of self-reported epilepsy in Canada. Epilepsia 2004;45:1623–9.

[2] Commission on Classification and Terminology of the International League Against Epilepsy. Proposal for revised clinical and electroencephalographic classification of epileptic seizures. Epilepsia 1981;22:489–501.

[3] Commission on Classification and Terminology of the International League Against Epilepsy. Proposal for classification of epilepsies and epileptic syndromes. Epilepsia 1985; 26:268–78.

[4] Lockman LA. Absence seizures and variants. Neurol Clin 1985;3:19–29.

[5] Wirrell EC. Natural history of absence epilepsy in children. Can J Neurol Sci 2003;30: 184–8.

[6] Wirrell EC, Camfield CS, Camfield PR, et al. IWK Hospital for Children H, Nova Scotia, Canada: long-term prognosis of typical childhood absence epilepsy: remission or progression to juvenile myoclonic epilepsy. Neurology 1996;47:912–8.

[7] Crunelli V, Leresche N. Childhood absence epilepsy: genes, channels, neurons and networks. Nat Rev Neurosci 2002;3:371–82.

[8] Ahmed S, Chadwick D, Walker RJ. The management of alcohol-related seizures: an overview. Hosp Med 2000;61:793–6.

[9] Ajmone-Marsan C, Zivin LS. Factors related to the occurrence of typical paroxysmal abnormalities in the EEG records of epileptic patients. Epilepsia 1970;11:361–81.

[10] Hauser WA, Anderson VE, Loewenson RB, et al. Seizure recurrence after a first unprovoked seizure. N Engl J Med 1982;307:522–8.

[11] Shinnar S, Berg AT, Moshe SL, et al. The risk of seizure recurrence after a first unprovoked afebrile seizure in childhoog: an extended follow-up. Pediatrics 1996;98(2 Pt 1):216–25.

[12] Renganathan R, Delanty N. Juvenile myoclonic epilepsy: under-appreciated and under-diagnosed. Postgrad Med J 2003;79:78–80.

[13] Genton P, Gelisse P. Juvenile myoclonic epilepsy. Arch Neurol 2001;58:1487–90.

[14] Delgado-Escueta AV, Enrile-Bacsal F. Juvenile myoclonic epilepsy of Janz. Neurology 1984; 34(3):285–94.

[15] Appleton R, Beirne M, Acomb B. Photosensitivity in juvenile myoclonic epilepsy. Seizure 2000;9:108–11.

[16] Badinand-Hubert N, Bureau M, Hirsch E, et al. Epilepsies and video games: results of a multicentric study. Electroencephalogr Clin Neurophysiol 1998;107:422–7.

[17] Kathare SV, Valencia I, Khurana DS, et al. Efficacy and tolerability of zonisamide in juvenile myoclonic epilepsy. Epileptic Disord 2004;6:267–70.

[18] Prasad A, Kuzniecky RI, Knowlton RC, et al. Evolving antiepileptic drug treatment in juvenile myclonic epilepsy. Arch Neurol 2003;60:1100–5.

[19] Buchanan N. The use of lamotrigine in juvenile myoclonic epilepsy. Seizure 1996;5:149–51.

[20] Carrazana EJ, Wheeler SD. Exacerbation of juvenile myoclonic epilepsy with lamotrigine. Neurology 2001;56:1424–5.

[21] Genton P, Gelisse P, Thomas P, et al. Do carbamazepine and phenytoin aggravate juvenile myoclonic epilepsy? Neurology 2000;55:1106–9.

[22] Snead OC, Hosey LC. Exacerbation of seizures in children by carbamazepine. N Engl J Med 1985;313:916–21.

[23] Kotagal P. Complex partial seizures with automatisms. In: Wyllie E, editor. The treatment of epilepsy: principles and practice. 2nd ed. Baltimore: Williams and Wilkins; 1997. p. 385–400.

[24] Rioux MH. Sterilization. Canadian Doctor 1979;45:66–8.

[25] Pennell PB. Pregnancy in women who have epilepsy. Neurol Clin 2004;22:799–820.

[26] Antiepileptics. Pregnancy and the child. Drug Ther Bull (England) 2005;43:13–6.

[27] Crawford P. Epilepsy and pregnancy. Seizure 2002;11(Suppl A):212–9.

[28] Wyszynski DF, Nambison M, Surve T, et al. Increased rate of malformations in offspring exposed to valproate during pregnancy. Neurology 2005;64:961–5.

[29] Tennis P, Eldridge RR. Preliminary results on pregnancy outcomes in women using lamotrigine. Epilepsia 2002;43:1161–7.

[30] Sabers A, Dam M, A-Rogvi-Hansen B, et al. Epilepsy and pregnancy: lamotrigine as main drug used. Acta Neurol Scand 2004;109:9–13.

[31] Cunnington MC. The International Lamotrigine pregnancy registry update for the epilepsy foundation. Epilepsia 2004;45:1468.

[32] Pennell PB, Newport DJ, Stowe ZN, et al. The impact of pregnancy and childbirth on the metabolism of lamotrigine. Neurology 2004;62:292–5.

[33] McKhann GM, Dourgeois BF, Goodman RR. Epilepsy surgery: indications, approaches, and results. Semin Neurol 2002;22:269–78.

[34] Shaefi S, Harkness W. Current status of surgery in the management of epilepsy. Epilepsia 2003;20:1195–215.

[35] Sheth RD. Epilepsy surgery. Presurgical evaluation. Neurol Clin 2002;20:1195–215.

[36] Tellez-Zenteno JF, Dhar R, Wiebe S. Long-term seizure outcomes following epilepsy surgery: a systematic review and meta-analysis. Brain 2005;128(Pt 5):188–98.

[37] Kwan P, Brodie MJ. Early identification of refractory epilepsy. N Engl J Med 2000;342: 314–9.

[38] Bergey GK. Minimizing misdiagnoses in epilepsy in the elderly. Geriatrics 2005;(Suppl): 12–9.

[39] Faught E. Epidemiology and drug treatment of epilepsy in elderly people. Drugs Aging 1999; 15:255–69.

[40] Hauser WA, Annegers JF, Kurland LT. Incidence of epilepsy and unprovoked seizures in Rochester, Minnesota: 1935–1984. Epilepsia 1993;34:453–68.

[41] Ruggles KH, Haessly SM, Berg RL. Prospective study of seizures in the elderly in the Marshfield Epidemiologic Study Area (MESA). Epilepsia 2001;42:1594–9.

[42] DeToledo JC. Changing presentation of seizures with aging: clinical and etiological factors. Gerontology 1999;45:329–35.

[43] Kellinghaus C, Loddenkemper T, Dinner DS, et al. Seizure semiology in the elderly: a video analysis. Epilepsia 2004;45:263–7.

[44] Ramsay RE, Rowan AJ, Pryor FM. Special considerations in treating the elderly patient with epilepsy. Neurology 2004;62(Suppl 2):S24–9.

[45] McBride AE, Shih TT, Hirsch LJ. Video-EEG monitoring in the elderly: a review of 94 patients. Epilepsia 2002;43:165–9.

[46] Hauser WA, Morris ML, Heston LL, et al. Seizures and myoclonus in patients with Alzheimer's disease. Neurology 1986;36:1226–30.

[47] Hesdorffer DC, Hauser WA, Annegers JF, et al. Dementia and adult-onset unprovoked seizures. Neurology 1996;46:727–30.

[48] Tiamkao S, Pratipanawatr T, Tiamkao S, et al. Seizures in non-ketotic hyperglycaemia. Seizure 2003;12:409–10.

[49] Willmore LJ. Antiepileptic drug therapy in the elderly. Pharmacol Ther 1998;78:9–16.

[50] Pugh MJ, Cramer J, Knoefel J, et al. Potentially inappropriate antiepileptic drugs for elderly patients with epilepsy. J Am Geriatr Soc 2004;52:417–22.

[51] Bergey GK. Initial treatment of epilepsy: special issues in treating the elderly. Neurology 2004;63(10, Suppl 4):S40–8.

[52] Leppik IE, Bergery GK, Ramsay RE, et al. Advances in epileptic drug treatment: a rational basis for selecting drugs for older people with epilepsy. Geriatrics 2004;59:14–8.

[53] Rowan AJ, Ramsay RE, Collins JF, et al. New onset geriatric epilepsy: a randomized study of gabapentin, lamotrigine, and carbamazepine. Neurology 2005;64:1868–73.

[54] Alsaadi TM, Koopmans S, Apperson M, et al. Levetiracetam monotherapy for elderly patients with epilepsy. Seizure 2004;13:58–60.

[55] Cramer JA, Leppik IE, Rue KD, et al. Tolerability of levetiracetam in elderly patients with CNS disorders. Epilepsy Res 2003;56:135–45.

ELSEVIER
SAUNDERS

Neurol Clin 24 (2006) 309–330

NEUROLOGIC
CLINICS

Spine Disorder Case Studies

J.D. Bartleson, MD

Department of Neurology, Mayo Clinic College of Medicine,
200 First Street, SW, Rochester, MN 55905, USA

Spine disorders causing spine and limb pain are extremely common. Fifteen to twenty percent of the United States population experiences low back pain (LBP) in a given year and among working age people, approximately 50% admit to back symptoms each year [1]. Neck and upper limb symptoms are somewhat less common but may be more worrisome because of concern that the spinal cord could be involved. Many health care providers are uncomfortable dealing with spine and limb pain because of the multiple possible causes; concern about potential loss of neurologic function; the cost of evaluating and treating these patients; and potential workers' compensation, legal, and medicolegal concerns. This article uses illustrative cases to describe the most common spine syndromes, when to consider additional investigation and consultation, and appropriate treatment options.

Patient 1—cervical radiculopathy

A 41-year-old, right-handed woman who keeps books for the family farm awoke 6 weeks previously with severe pain in her right posterior shoulder. The pain soon spread into her right elbow and forearm, and she noted a funny feeling in her right forefinger and weakness of extension of her right elbow. The symptoms fluctuated but overall have been worsening, and the pain wakes her from sleep at night. She has had no difficulty with use of her lower limbs and no trouble with bowel or bladder function. She has been taking hydrocodone with acetaminophen with partial pain control. Medical history is significant only for a successful lumbar laminectomy and discectomy for low back and right lower limb pain a decade ago. Neurologic examination is significant for severe weakness in the right C7 distribution with reduction of the right triceps reflex and a normal sensory examination.

E-mail address: bartleson.john@mayo.edu

0733-8619/06/$ - see front matter © 2006 Elsevier Inc. All rights reserved.
doi:10.1016/j.ncl.2006.01.004
neurologic.theclinics.com

How would this patient be evaluated and treated? She has a right C7 radiculopathy, which began rather acutely. Although not as common as lumbar radiculopathy, cervical radiculopathy has a reported annual incidence rate of 107.3 per 100,000 men and 63.5 per 100,000 women (total annual incidence 83.2 per 100,000) with a peak between the ages of 50 and 54 [2]. Only 15% of cases have a history of head and neck trauma, whereas 41% have a history of lumbar radiculopathy. Radiculopathy is defined as dysfunction of a spinal nerve, the roots of the nerve, or both and usually presents with pain in the spine and limb (or trunk in the case of thoracic radiculopathy), sensory disturbance, weakness, or reflex reduction in the appropriate distribution.

The natural history of cervical radiculopathy is that of improvement with medical or surgical treatment, but one third of patients experience recurrence during a median follow-up of 4.9 years [2]. Ninety percent of patients have no symptoms or only mild incapacitation with longer follow-up.

The most frequent cause of cervical radiculopathy is compression of the spinal nerve in the foramen where it leaves the cervical spine resulting from a combination of factors, including degenerative, hypertrophic changes of the uncovertebral joints and zygapophyseal joints or herniation of the intervertebral nucleus pulposus [2,3]. Other causes include tumors, trauma, and infectious and noninfectious inflammatory conditions.

Signs and symptoms associated with cervical radiculopathy depend on the level of involvement (Table 1). Because there are eight numbered cervical roots and only seven cervical vertebra and the intervertebral foramina and disks are numbered according to the vertebra above, the cervical nerve root involved is one number higher than the disk level. Thus, a C7 radiculopathy is the result of neural compression at or near the C6-7 foramen. With cervical spondylosis, C7 root compression is most common, followed by C6 radiculopathy, C8 radiculopathy, and C5 radiculopathy.

The differential diagnosis of potentially neurogenic upper limb pain includes peripheral nerve entrapment, disorders of the rotator cuff and shoulder, brachial plexus neuritis, thoracic outlet syndrome, herpes zoster, Pancoast's syndrome, complex regional pain syndrome, and referred somatic pain from the neck [3]. The diagnosis of cervical radiculopathy can be made or strongly suspected from the history and physical and neurologic examinations. Similar to the situation for LBP, clinicians should be on the lookout for red flags in patient history, which include trauma (for possible fracture); age over 50 or under 20, past history of cancer, fever or chills unexplained weight loss, recent bacterial infection, intravenous drug use, immunosuppression from any cause, pain that worsens when the patient is supine (possible tumor or infection); and a severe or progressive neurologic deficit. The presence of any red flag should increase the index of suspicion and lead to earlier and more thorough investigation. Additionally, ask about symptoms of myelopathy and look for evidence of myelopathy on neurologic examination, the presence of which influences the timing of

Table 1
Symptoms and signs associated with cervical radiculopathy

Root	Pain distribution	Dermatomal sensory distribution	Weakness	Affected reflex
C4	Upper neck	"Cape" distribution shoulder/arm	Usually none	None
C5	Neck, scapula, shoulder, anterior arm	Lateral aspect of arm and forearm	Shoulder abduction Forearm flexion Forearm pronation	Biceps Brachioradialis
C6	Neck, scapula, shoulder, lateral arm and forearm, and thumb and forefinger	Lateral aspect of forearm and hand and thumb and forefinger	Shoulder abduction Forearm flexion	Biceps Brachioradialis
C7	Neck, shoulder, lateral arm, medial scapula, extensor surface of forearm	Dorsolateral forearm and hand, forefinger and long finger	Elbow extension Wrist extension Finger extension	Triceps
C8	Neck, medial scapula, medial aspect arm and forearm, and ring and little fingers	Medial forearm and hand and ring and little fingers	Finger abduction Finger adduction Finger flexors	Finger flexors

Adapted from Levin KH, Covington ED, Devereaux MW, et al. Neck and back pain. Continuum 2001;7(1):15; with permission.

testing and treatment recommendations. Signs and symptoms of myelopathy are listed in Box 1 and described in greater detail later.

Patient 1 clearly has a C7 radiculopathy and no reason to suspect anything more worrisome than cervical spondylosis. Which, if any, tests are appropriate? Routine laboratory studies are not recommended [3]. Plain radiographs of the cervical spine likewise are unnecessary [3].

MRI is the test of choice to confirm spondylotic nerve root compression and exclude more sinister causes. In the absence of red flags or signs or symptoms of myelopathy, a recent review states, "it is appropriate to limit the use of MRI to those remaining symptomatic after four to six weeks of nonsurgical treatment" [3]. CT scan alone is less helpful, but CT myelography is useful as an alternative and sometimes as a complement to MRI.

Electromyography (EMG) and nerve conduction studies can be helpful in documenting radiculopathy, but changes may not be evident for 3 to 4 weeks after the onset of nerve injury. When the diagnosis of a single radiculopathy is clear, as in Patient 1, there is no need for EMG. EMG can be helpful in confirming that the problem is a cervical radiculopathy and not a brachial plexopathy or more peripheral nerve lesion, differentiating neurogenic from non-neurogenic pain, determining if the radiculopathy is old or new, and helping to localize the spinal level involved if the signs and

---

Box 1. Symptoms and signs of myelopathy

Symptoms associated with myelopathy
Neck and unilateral or bilateral upper limb pain
Upper limb weakness, numbness, or loss of dexterity
Lower limb stiffness, weakness, or sensory loss
Urgency of bladder more often than bowel, urgency
   incontinence, frequency of urination
Lhermitte's sign (shock-like sensations extending down the spine
   and out into the limbs with neck flexion)

Findings associated with myelopathy
Increased lower or upper limb deep tendon reflexes
Positive Hoffmann's (thumb adduction and flexion and finger
   flexion after forced flexion and sudden release of the tip of the
   long finger)
Babinski's signs
Upper limb weakness beyond the bounds of a single nerve root
   on one or both sides
Weakness in the lower limbs in an upper motor neuron
   distribution
Sensory loss
Spasticity in the limbs, especially the lower extremities
Gait disturbance, especially if suggestive of spasticity

---

symptoms or imaging leave room for doubt. These same comments apply to patients who have acute or chronic lumbar radiculopathy.

Nonsurgical management should be the first line of treatment for most patients who have cervical radiculopathy. None of the recommended treatments have been subjected to randomized, placebo-controlled trials, and patient preference should be considered [3]. Analgesics, including nonsteroidal anti-inflammatory drugs (NSAIDs), acetaminophen, and opioids for severe pain, can be used. Anecdotal reports of a 1-week course of tapering oral steroids and translaminar and transforaminal epidural corticosteroid injections note benefit, but the injections in particular can have serious side effects. It is difficult to judge the response because many patients improve spontaneously [2]. Physical measures, including short-term intermittent or continuous use of a cervical collar, heat or ice, and intermittent cervical traction, are all used. Neck exercises can be used as patient pain allows.

Is surgery helpful for patients who have persistent cervical radiculopathy? A Cochrane review found a single prospective, randomized trial that reports that surgical treatment for spondylotic cervical radiculopathy was more helpful than physical therapy or a cervical collar 3 to 4 months after intervention, but outcomes were the same at 1 year [4,5]. Generally accepted indications for surgical intervention for cervical radiculopathy include persistent pain in the upper extremity lasting 4 to 6 weeks or longer with strong physiologic evidence of dysfunction of a specific cervical nerve root and confirmation of nerve root impingement at the appropriate level and side on an imaging study. Factors that can influence the referral and operative decision include a progressive radicular deficit, any signs or symptoms of spinal cord impingement, a larger-sized herniated disk on the imaging study, profound pain, or weakness that is critical to a patient's vocation or avocation.

Surgery for spondylotic radiculopathy can be performed from a posterior approach in which part of the lamina on one side is removed, and the offending bony spurs or protruding intervertebral disk are cut out. Alternatively, surgery can be performed from an anterior approach in which the appropriate intervertebral disk is removed and either autologous or cadaver bone or synthetic materials are implanted, and often plates and screws are placed permanently into the two adjacent vertebral bodies to promote bony fusion. The two approaches have comparable results, with approximately 75% of patients experiencing substantial relief from their radicular symptoms [5–7]. Complications occur in a small percentage of patients and include nerve root more likely than spinal cord injury and hoarseness and swallowing difficulty after anterior cervical spine surgery. Both procedures are performed by neurosurgeons and orthopedic surgeons.

Because of the lack of clear-cut evidence that surgical treatment is superior to medical management, surgery for cervical radiculopathy should be considered elective. Patient 1 was found to have a large right C6-7 paracentral disk protrusion that flattened the spinal cord mildly and caused severe right C6-7 neural foraminal narrowing with C7 nerve root compression. She elected to have surgery, underwent posterior cervical laminectomy and discectomy, and experienced prompt relief of pain and gradual, good recovery of motor function.

Patient 2—cervical spondylotic myelopathy

A 72-year-old man presented with a 6-month history of worsening unsteadiness when walking. He also noted some clumsiness with use of his upper limbs and some frequency and mild urgency of urination. He reported no pain and had no cognitive difficulty. Examination showed a mildly spastic-ataxic gait, weakness in both hands and in both lower limbs in an upper motor neuron distribution, decreased joint position and vibration sense in the lower limbs, generalized hyperreflexia, and bilateral Hoffmann's and Babinski's signs.

This patient clearly had evidence of a myelopathy localized to the cervical level. The differential diagnosis of cervical myelopathy is lengthy (Box 2). The most common cause for myelopathy, especially in individuals at or beyond middle age, is cervical spondylosis. The condition is associated

Box 2. Differential diagnosis of cervical myelopathy

Causes of cervical myelopathy with canal stenosis
Acquired
  Cervical spondylosis
  Paget disease
  Fluorosis
  Ossification of posterior longitudinal ligament
  Diffuse idiopathic skeletal hyperostosis
  Cervical disk herniation
  Rheumatoid arthritis or ankylosing spondylitis with upper
    cervical subluxation
  Fracture
  Gout
Congenital
  Multiple hereditary exostoses
  Maroteaux-Lamy syndrome
  Achondroplasia

Causes of cervical myelopathy without canal stenosis
  Cervical spine tumor; intramedullary, extramedullary,
    extradural
  Syringomyelia
  Arteriovenous malformation
  Multiple sclerosis
  Amyotrophic lateral sclerosis
  Subacute combined degeneration (vitamin B_{12} deficiency)
  Neurosyphilis
  Hereditary spastic paraparesis
  Human T-lymphotropic virus-1 (HTLV-1) or HIV infection
  Adrenoleukodystrophy
  Parasagittal cerebral lesion, such as tumor
  Multiple strokes, brainstem stroke
  Spinal cord infarction
  Transverse myelitis
  Radiation myelopathy
  Neurosarcoidosis
  Autoimmune diseases, including vasculitis
  Paraneoplastic syndrome
  Copper deficiency

Adapted from Bartleson JD, O'Duffy JD. Spinal stenosis. In: Koopman WJ,
editor. Arthritis and allied conditions. 14th ed. Baltimore: Lippincott Williams &
Wilkins; 2001. p. 2044; with permission.

with degenerative and hypertrophic changes, usually of the lower cervical spine and especially if the changes are superimposed on a spinal canal that is narrowed congenitally from front to back. Men outnumber women in a ratio of 3:2 [8].

The presentation is variable and depends on the predominance of motor versus sensory symptoms, upper versus lower limb symptoms, changes in muscle tone, upper versus lower motor neuron phenomena in the upper extremities, and sphincter complaints (see Box 1). In decreasing order, patients have abnormal reflexes; spasticity; gait difficulty; frequency and urgency of urination; sensory symptoms, including proprioceptive loss; and (less commonly) paresthesias, radicular upper limb pain, and neck pain [8,9]. As with Patient 2, the condition can be painless.

Depending on the level and degree of compression, there may be lower or upper motor neuron signs in the upper extremities and, therefore, the upper limb reflexes can be decreased or increased, especially the triceps reflex. Lower motor neuron findings with weakness and wasting in the hand and forearm muscles are common. The lower motor neuron findings in the upper limbs and some of the upper extremity sensory symptoms can be the result of cervical radiculopathy, and cervical spondylotic myeloradiculopathy is a more appropriate term than myelopathy for most patients who have this condition. Patients may report Lhermitte's phenomenon. Patients may report sudden worsening after a neck injury, which can be mild, especially with one involving sudden flexion or extension. The spinal cord findings can be asymmetric, and the patient can present with a partial Brown-Séquard syndrome.

Which tests should be obtained in Patient 2? MRI again is the diagnostic test of choice and can help exclude many of the other possibilities in the differential diagnosis. If MRI is not possible, then myelography with CT scan is recommended. Myelography with CT scanning can demonstrate increased spinal cord compression with neck extension, which is not feasible with MRI. Cervical spondylotic myelopathy frequently is a multilevel process. MRI has the advantage of showing abnormal T2 signal within the cervical spinal cord, which is believed to indicate that the spinal cord compression is significant [7]. Plain CT and plain radiographs of the cervical spine have limited usefulness. MRI of the brain and thoracolumbar spine can help exclude other possibilities in the differential diagnosis. EMG can help exclude motor neuron disease and brachial plexus and peripheral nerve disease. Blood tests can help exclude vitamin B_{12} deficiency, HTLV-1 and HIV infection, syphilis, and copper deficiency [10] as causes of myelopathy. Cervical spondylosis is common, if not universal with aging, and some degree of cervical spinal stenosis with apparent mild spinal cord compression can be asymptomatic, and, thus, clinical correlation between patients' signs and symptoms and radiographic findings is imperative.

Patient 2's MRI scan showed significant cervical spinal canal stenosis and spinal cord compression at C6-7 more than C5-6 with some increased T2 signal within the spinal cord. Which treatment should be recommended? Should surgery be suggested? Although some patients who have spondylotic myelopathy remain stable for several years with conservative treatment [11,12], a substantial number of patients do worsen over time, sometimes fairly suddenly, and spontaneous improvement in the neurologic signs and symptoms is rare. Conservative treatment consists of the use of a cervical collar and physical therapy directed at a patient's neurologic problems.

Although there is consensus that surgical decompression is indicated at least for patients who have moderate or worse deficits and for progressive neurologic symptoms [7–9,13,14], a Cochrane review regarding surgery for cervical myelopathy [4] could find only a single randomized trial of 49 patients comparing surgery with conservative treatment for cervical spondylotic myelopathy, which showed no significant difference in outcome [15], which also was true for a more recent study of 68 patients [16]. The paucity of studies no doubt relates to the strongly held belief that surgical intervention is helpful.

As is the case with cervical radiculopathy, surgical decompression can be performed from in front using discectomy with interbody fusion or from a posterior approach with bilateral laminectomy or laminoplasty. Anterior decompression and fusion are favored in patients who have instability of the spine or stenosis confined to one or two levels, whereas the posterior approach may be favored in patients who have compression at two or more levels. With either approach, approximately 70% of patients experience initial improvement, but some experience later gradual deterioration even in the absence of recurrent compression [8,9,13]. Patient 2 underwent two-level posterior decompression with good but incomplete improvement in his neurologic signs and symptoms.

Patient 3—lumbar radiculopathy

A 39-year-old male attorney reported a 1-month history of low back and left posterolateral thigh and leg pain, which began after a weekend of gardening. Initially, the back pain was worse, but then the left lower limb pain predominated, and he noted a "slapping" of his left foot when he walked and some numbness and tingling of his left foot. Aside from two prior bouts of LBP alone in the past and ongoing cigarette smoking, the patient's medical history was unrevealing. Examination showed moderately severe weakness in the left L5 distribution. Lower limb reflexes were normal and symmetric, sensory examination was normal, and straight-leg raising aggravated the patient's pain at 30° elevation on the left.

Low back problems are common and second to upper respiratory problems as a symptom-related reason for seeing a health care provider [1,17,18].

LBP can be caused by many different pathophysiologic mechanisms, and perhaps 85% of patients who have isolated LBP cannot be given a precise pathoanatomic diagnosis [17]. The peak prevalence for LBP is between the ages of 30 and 55, and there is little difference between men and women. Risk factors include heavy lifting and twisting, vibration of the body, prolonged sitting or standing, monotonous work, job dissatisfaction, and poor relationships with coworkers [17]. Smoking is a weak, but definite, risk factor for disk degeneration and LBP [19]. There is marked variation in the use of diagnostic tests and treatments, especially surgery, for patients who have LBP between countries and between regions within the United States [17]. Work-related and non–work-related injuries and medicolegal factors complicate the care of patients who have back pain. For those under age 45, low back problems are the most common cause of disability; approximately 1% of the United States population is disabled chronically by back pain and another 1% temporarily unable to work at any one time [1]. For all of these reasons, the evaluation and treatment of patients who have LBP can be difficult and frustrating for patients and providers and can lead to excessive investigation and inappropriate treatment.

Fortunately, the natural history of acute low back with and without radiation into the lower limb is benign, with 90% of patients reporting gradual resolution over the course of 1 week to a month or 2. Patients who have accompanying lower limb pain tend to improve somewhat more slowly than patients who have LBP alone. Recurrences are common, and perhaps 10% of patients go on to experience chronic pain.

Deyo and Weinstein divide the differential diagnosis of LBP broadly into mechanical low back or leg pain (no underlying neoplastic or inflammatory disease), nonmechanical spinal conditions (neoplasia, infections, and inflammatory arthritis), and visceral disease of the pelvic and intra-abdominal organs, which they estimate account for approximately 97%, 1%, and 2% of cases, respectively [17]. The major sources of low back and lower limb pain are listed in Box 3.

The job of clinicians is to make sure that there are no worrisome symptoms or findings that should prompt additional investigation and, if there are none, to treat patients conservatively while watching for the emergence of those symptoms and findings. The so-called "red flags" for potentially serious conditions causing LBP with referred lower limb pain are similar to those for cervical radiculopathy (Table 2). It especially is important to recognize the development of an acute or subacute cauda equina syndrome (CES). Clinical features can include perineal and other lumbosacral root sensory deficits, lower limb motor weakness, difficulty with bladder more often than bowel control, sexual dysfunction, LBP, and unilateral or bilateral sciatica. There is evidence from a meta-analysis that surgical decompression within 48 hours of onset of CES resulting from a large lumbar disk herniation improves outcomes [20]. CES should be evaluated and treated very urgently, if not emergently. If there are no red flags and, thus, no suspicion of underlying cancer, infection, fracture, or significant neurologic compromise, then no diagnostic studies are recommended for the first month after onset of LBP [1,17,18,21].

Box 3. Major sources of low back and lower limb pain

Musculoskeletal affecting the spine, pelvis, and lower limbs
Joint
Disk
Bone
Muscle
Ligament, tendon, and other soft tissue

Neurogenic
Central nervous system (lower spinal cord)
Nerve root
Lumbosacral plexus
Peripheral nerve
Meninges

Viscerogenic
Pancreas
Bowel
Kidney
Ureter
Bladder
Uterus
Ovary
Prostate

Vascular
Abdominal aortic aneurysm
Atherosclerotic peripheral vascular disease

Psychogenic
With an additional source of pain
Rarely, without an additional source

Turning to Patient 3, what is his diagnosis? Pain in the sciatic nerve distribution is the single most useful history item indicating disk herniation [22]. Additionally, the patient had clear-cut evidence of an L5 distribution motor deficit. The typical symptoms and signs associated with lumbosacral radiculopathies are shown in Table 3. EMG is unnecessary because the patient has a clinically obvious L5 radiculopathy. There are no red flags to suggest tumor, infection, occult fracture, or CES, and any additional investigation can be deferred at this time. The patient did have moderately severe weakness, however, and imaging to confirm the presence of a disk, assess its size, and rule out more serious causes is reasonable at this juncture. MRI is the diagnostic imaging test of choice, but CT myelography or even

Table 2
Red flags for potentially serious conditions causing low back pain

Possible fracture	Major trauma, such as motor vehicle accident or fall from height
	Minor trauma or lifting a weight in an older or potentially osteoporotic patient
Possible tumor or infection	Age >50 or <20
	History of cancer
	Recent fever or chills or unexplained weight loss
	Recent bacterial infection, intravenous drug abuse or immunosuppression
	Pain that worsens when supine or wakes patient from sleep at night
Possible CES	History or examination evidence of perianal/perineal sensory loss
	Recent onset of bladder or bowel dysfunction or unexpected weakness of anal sphincter on examination
	History of severe or progressive lower limb neurologic deficit
	Major lower limb motor weakness on examination

Adapted from Bigos SJ, Bowyer OR, Braen GR, et al. Acute low back problems in adults. Clinical practice guideline and quick reference guide, number 14. Rockville (MD): US Department of Health and Human Services, Public Health Service, Agency for Health Care Policy and Research; December 1994. AHCPR publication number 95-0642 and 95-0643.

plain CT could be chosen. Clinical correlation is important because approximately one third of asymptomatic volunteers show evidence of one or more herniated intervertebral lumbar disks [23]. Blood tests are not needed given the absence of any indication of systemic illness.

Table 3
Symptoms and signs associated with lumbar radiculopathy

Root	Pain distribution	Dermatomal sensory distribution	Weakness	Affected reflex
L1	Inguinal region	Inguinal region	Hip flexion	Cremasteric
L2	Inguinal region and anterior thigh	Anterior thigh	Hip flexion Hip adduction	Cremasteric Thigh adductor
L3	Anterior thigh and knee	Distal anteromedial thigh, including knee	Knee extension Hip flexion Hip adduction	Patellar Thigh adductor
L4	Anterior thigh, medial aspect leg	Medial leg	Knee extension Hip flexion Hip adduction	Patellar
L5	Posterolateral thigh Lateral leg Medial foot	Lateral leg, dorsal foot, and great toe	Foot dorsiflexion Knee flexion Hip abduction	Possibly internal hamstring
S1	Posterior thigh and leg and lateral foot	Posterolateral leg and lateral aspect of foot	Foot plantar flexion Knee flexion Hip extension	Achilles

Adapted from Levin KH, Covington ED, Devereaux MW, et al. Neck and back pain. Continuum 2001;7(1);16; with permission.

As expected, this patient's MRI scan showed a significant lumbar disk protrusion at L4-5 on the left. Although the L5 nerve root exits the spine underneath the L5 pedicle, this is lateral to and often slightly above the L5-S1 interspace; unless a disk protrusion is quite far lateral, it will, in general, affect the nerve root one segment below the level of protrusion. Thus, L4 disk protrusion usually is responsible for L5 nerve root impingement as the L5 root migrates laterally before exiting below the L5 pedicle. More than 90% of disk herniations occur at L4-5 (and produce L5 radiculopathy) and L5-S1 (and cause S1 radiculopathy) [1,18]. Herniations at L3-4 (with L4 radiculopathy) and L2-3 (with L3 radiculopathy) are less common. Large and lateral disk protrusions can affect the root at the same level as the disk herniation, and large disk herniations can compress more than one root on one side and, if large enough, can cause bilateral lumbosacral root compression and the CES.

How should this patient and other patients who have acute LBP and lumbar radiculopathy be treated? Bed rest is not recommended; patients are advised to be up and about as their pain allows [17,24,25]. Analgesics, in particular NSAIDs, and acetaminophen can be used as comfort control measures [1,17,21,25,26]. Muscle relaxants also can be helpful for patients who have acute LBP but have side effects [25,27]. Opioid analgesics can be used on a time-limited basis [1,21]. Injections of corticosteroids, usually with a local anesthetic given epidurally or transforaminally, are an option for short-term relief of radicular pain if conservative measures fail and as a means of trying to avoid surgery [1,25]. Although commonly used, evidence is lacking for the use of epidural injections for acute and subacute LBP without radiculopathy [1,25,28]. Spinal manipulation and physical therapy can be used in patients who have acute or subacute LBP, but the benefits are limited and many patients recover without intervention [17].

Should this patient have surgery for his lumbar disk protrusion? Presuming that the patient did not have fracture with instability, infection that requires culture or drainage, tumor that requires biopsy or removal, or CES, which should be decompressed urgently, the indications for lumbar radiculopathy, which are similar to those for cervical radiculopathy, are as follows. The patient should have sciatica in addition to LBP; the patient's sciatica should be severe and disabling; the pain or associated neurologic deficits should have persisted without improvement for more than 4 weeks or progressed during observation; and there should be strong physiologic evidence for dysfunction of a specific nerve root with confirmation of disk herniation at the appropriate level on an imaging study [1,17,18,21,29]. Weakness that is critical to the patient's job or favored leisure activity can influence the surgical decision. Sometimes with lumbar and cervical radiculopathy, there can be worsening of the neurologic deficit associated with lessening limb or spine pain resulting from increased nerve root compression.

Laminectomy and lumbar discectomy can relieve symptoms quicker than nonsurgical medical and physical therapies in patients who have significant radicular symptoms who have not improved after 1 to 2 months of conservative treatment. Evidence shows that discectomy provides better pain relief than nonoperative treatment for up to 4 years, although there is no clear advantage 10 years after surgery [17,21,30,31].

Patient 3 elected an epidural steroid injection, which helped his pain. Six months later, he had only mild LBP and moderate, improving left L5 distribution weakness, which did not interfere with his work or leisure activities.

Patient 4—lumbar spinal stenosis

A 76-year-old man reported a 1-year history of increasing LBP and bilateral, posterior, lower limb pain and weakness with standing and walking. It helped to walk behind a cart. He had no symptoms when sitting or lying down. He had a history of hypertension, prior coronary artery bypass grafting, and mild angina pectoris. Neurologic examination showed only loss of vibration sense in the toes and absence of the ankle reflexes.

This patient was describing pseudoclaudication and mostly likely had lumbar spinal stenosis (LSS) defined as narrowing of the lumbar spinal canal, its lateral recesses, or neural foramina with associated compression of the lumbosacral nerve roots. The precise incidence and prevalence of this condition are not known, but LSS increases with age and is a common problem. Men and women are affected approximately equally. Although disability and pain control issues are less frequent with LSS than with acute and chronic LBP, the impact on quality of life is roughly the same [8,18,32–35].

LSS can be the result of congenital or acquired causes. Any of the structures that surround the lumbar spinal canal can hypertrophy and lead to narrowing of the lumbar spinal canal. Often there are degenerative changes superimposed on a congenitally narrow spinal canal. Facet joint hypertrophy is the leading cause of LSS with contributions from disk degeneration, vertebral body hypertrophy, thickening and bulging of the ligamentum flavum, and degenerative spondylolisthesis. In descending order, the most commonly affected levels are L4-5, L3-4, L2-3, L5-S1, and L1-2. Most patients have narrowing at more than one level. Spinal canal narrowing can be asymmetric or affect the lateral recess or neural foramen on one side and, thus, can result in asymmetric or unilateral symptoms [8,18].

The majority of patients who have LSS have a remote history of LBP, and approximately one fifth have a history of sciatica. In general, LSS is a chronic and gradually progressive condition, but rare patients report spontaneous improvement. The hallmark of LSS is neurogenic or so-called "pseudoclaudication." Patients report pain, numbness, tingling, or weakness in the lower limbs typically brought on by standing and walking and relieved by sitting or flexing forward at the waist [8,18,34,35]. Postures that maintain or increase lumbar flexion, such as walking behind a cart or lawn mower, using a stationary bicycle, or leaning against an object, help to prevent or relieve pseudoclaudication. Conversely, activities that increase lumbar lordosis, such as wearing higher-heeled shoes or walking down an incline, can increase symptoms. In advanced cases, patients may experience symptoms when recumbent. Pseudoclaudication often is variable and may be influenced by time of day, total time spent on the feet, floor surface, or nothing [8,18,34].

There are few physical findings on examination, and none are diagnostic. Deep tendon reflexes are reduced at the ankle in approximately half of patients and at the knee in approximately one fourth [34]. Fixed unilateral or bilateral deficits, often in an L5 or S1 distribution, can be found in approximately one third of patients and are more likely to occur if patients have an underlying peripheral neuropathy. Straight-leg raising typically is negative. Foot pulses should be normal unless there is co-existing atherosclerotic occlusive disease.

A differential diagnosis of pseudoclaudication is shown in Table 4. Multiple sclerosis and arteriovenous malformations of the spinal cord can cause pseudoclaudication-like symptoms. In patients who have multiple sclerosis, the exertion involved with walking can raise their body temperature slightly and cause a Uhthoff's phenomenon with the development of temporary lower limb numbness or weakness that resolves with rest. Although uncommon, spinal cord vascular malformations also can cause pseudoclaudication-like symptoms. Dural arteriovenous fistulas (DAVF) are the most common spinal cord vascular malformation and often present with symmetric or asymmetric sensory loss, lower limb weakness, and sometimes pain in the low back and lower limbs that can worsen with standing, walking, and Valsalva's maneuver [36]. DAVF affect middle-aged and older men more often than women, and it is believed that high-pressure arterial flow from a radicular artery causes venous hypertension, engorgement, and secondary spinal cord ischemia. The large majority of DAVF involve the thoracolumbar spinal cord. Subtle evidence of myelopathy on

Table 4
Differential diagnosis of lumbar stenosis

Vascular claudication—usually resulting from atherosclerotic disease
Osteoarthritis of hips or knees
Lumbar disk protrusion
Unrecognized neurologic disease
  Multiple sclerosis
  Intraspinal tumor
  Spinal cord arteriovenous malformations
  Peripheral neuropathy
  Rarely, communicating hydrocephalus

Adapted from Bartleson JD, O'Duffy JD. Spinal stenosis. In: Koopman WJ, editor. Arthritis and allied conditions. 14th ed. Baltimore: Lippincott Williams & Wilkins; 2001. p. 2048; with permission.

examination often is encountered; bowel and bladder dysfunction usually occurs relatively late [36]. EMG can be normal or show polyradiculopathy or even anterior horn cell disease. MRI with and without gadolinium is the diagnostic test of choice, but the spinal cord also must be imaged. MRI in DAVF shows areas of intramedullary increased T2 signal in the spinal cord with patchy, diffuse spinal cord enhancement often with significant, enlarged pial blood vessels. Myelography with CT scanning sometimes is used to help confirm the presence of serpiginous blood vessels on the surface of the spinal cord. Spinal magnetic resonance angiography is used to confirm the presence of a DAVF and guide the performance of conventional catheter spinal angiography, which can define the abnormal vascular anatomy and help plan surgical intervention. Surgical disconnection of the DAVF reverses the pathophysiology and, especially if performed early in the course, can result in symptomatic improvement [36].

If the diagnosis of LSS is clear and patients and providers agree that no intervention is needed at this time, investigation can be deferred. MRI is the imaging procedure of choice to diagnose LSS; plain CT or myelography with CT scanning also can be used. Asymptomatic central canal LSS is seen in approximately 5% of middle-aged and older adults [37], and clinicians must ensure that patient symptoms are consistent with the imaging findings. Vascular laboratory evaluation can confirm or exclude lower limb atherosclerotic disease. Plain films of the lumbosacral spine are nondiagnostic but can show dense bony structures, degenerative disk disease, and degenerative spondylolisthesis, which is seen frequently and typically affects L4 on L5. Plain radiographs of the hips or knees can determine if arthritis of these joints is contributing to symptoms. EMG usually shows changes consistent with lumbosacral nerve root injury and helps to exclude peripheral neuropathy, but a normal EMG does not exclude LSS [8,18,34].

Therapy for LSS can be divided into physical, pharmacologic, and surgical categories. Exercises to strengthen the abdominal muscles and reduce lumbar lordosis may be helpful. The use of a short cane or rolling walker may allow patients to stand longer and walk farther. Corsets and braces may help reduce lumbar lordosis when standing, thereby delaying the onset the symptoms. Much of the excess weight in obese patients is carried in their abdomen, forcing them to extend their lumbar spine to maintain their balance. Substantial weight loss can help relieve the symptoms of LSS by reducing the degree of lumbar extension (lordosis) needed to stand erect and by reducing the axial load on the lumbar spine [8,18].

Analgesics are not usually helpful, because the patient's pain is intermittent and can be relieved by sitting or lying down. NSAIDs and acetaminophen are preferred over opioid analgesics. Muscle relaxants are of no benefit. Epidural steroid injections may provide temporary pain relief but sometimes are difficult to perform because of the accompanying degenerative changes and canal stenosis [1,35,38].

Surgical decompression is the most effective treatment for LSS, which may need to be coupled with fusion if there is preoperative or the potential for postoperative spondylolisthesis with instability [1,8,32–35]. Patients often require decompression of more than one spinal level and may require foraminotomies and removal of one or more facet joints to provide lateral decompression. LBP, even if it is postural and accompanies the pseudoclaudication symptoms, may or may not improve after surgery. Surgery is, in general, not recommended for patients who have postural LBP associated with LSS if they do not have associated pseudoclaudication [1,8,18,35].

Because of increased recognition of LSS, the availability of CT and MRI scanning of the spine, and the increasing age of the United States population, there has been a marked increase in the rate of surgery for LSS in recent decades [39]. Factors associated with complications and disappointing results from surgery for LSS include age of the patient, absence of appropriate indications, performing fusion with decompression, increase in mechanical LBP after surgery, and comorbidities—other medical problems that increase the risk of operating and limit patients' functional ability and survival [39,40].

Because of the risk of complications, the unpredictable outcome of surgery, and the intermittency of symptoms, surgery for LSS is elective. In a 7- to 10-year follow-up of patients who underwent decompressive surgery for LSS, Katz and colleagues found that 23% had undergone reoperation for recurrent back and lower limb symptoms and 33% had severe LBP, but 75% were satisfied with the results of their initial surgery [41].

Patient 4 elected an epidural steroid injection, which did reduce his symptoms for approximately 2 months. Currently, he is taking a wait-and-see approach and using a four-wheeled rolling walker with hand brakes, seat, and basket.

Patient 5—chronic low back pain

A 47-year-old, right-handed farmer reported that he has had LBP "all of my life." He has had ups and downs through the years, but now he has been in a persistent flare-up for nearly 1 year. Nothing seemed to set off the increase in his LBP, which was in the middle of his lumbar spine and extended out a few inches to both sides. Sometimes when sitting, he had pain into his buttocks. Aside from cigarette smoking, he otherwise was in good health. Neurologic and musculoskeletal examinations essentially were normal. He already had plain radiographs and an MRI of the lumbar spine, which showed moderate degenerative disk and facet joint disease throughout the lumbar spine, most severe at the L4-5 interspace where the disk space was narrowed, and the MRI showed signal change abnormalities in the vertebral bodies adjacent to the degenerated L4-5 disk. Ibuprofen was of some benefit, whereas an epidural steroid injection provided no help.

Persistent LBP can be problematic for providers and patients. The frequency of the problem, multiplicity of causes, and the diagnostic approach were discussed previously. LBP without sciatica or stenosis is reported to have a point prevalence as high as 33% and a 1-year prevalence as high as 73% [42].

Evaluation depends on patient age and presentation. Testing depends specifically on the duration and intensity of pain, whether or not the pain is worsening or improving, the presence of associated signs and symptoms, the results of prior testing, and provider suspicions [17,18,21,42]. Red flags are similar to those for acute LBP (see Table 2) [1,17,18,21,42]. Deyo and Weinstein [17] recommend addressing the following three questions:

1. Is a systemic disease causing the pain?
2. Are there social or psychologic factors that may be amplifying or prolonging the pain?
3. Is there neurologic compromise that may require surgical evaluation and intervention?

For most patients, red flags can be determined and these three questions answered after a careful history and physical and neurologic examinations. Although they are not always necessary, many patients who have chronic LBP undergo imaging studies, usually plain radiographs and MRI. Again, care is needed in the interpretation because with age, degenerative changes in the lumbar spine are ubiquitous. Plain films can be used to screen for spondylolisthesis. Additional diagnostic studies used in patients who have persistent disabling LBP include provocative injections (discography) and anesthetic blockade in an attempt to identify a pain generator [42]. These diagnostic studies are imperfect at best, carry some small risk, and are left best to spine specialists who are evaluating patients for possible invasive surgery.

Psychosocial issues can increase the severity and duration of pain and reduce the benefits of attempted treatment. Although they need to be taken into account when assessing and treating patients, the psychosocial factors themselves are difficult to address. Patient 5 had no evidence of a systemic disease and, fortunately, did not seem to have any social or psychologic distress that could be influencing his pain. He had no neurologic symptoms or signs, and his imaging did not show any neural compression. This patient had severe lumbar spondylosis, especially at L4-5, which is presumed to be the source of his back pain. What treatment can be offered to this patient and others in whom there is less certainty that their pain is related to imaging findings?

Drug treatment includes analgesics, anti-inflammatory drugs, muscle relaxants, tricyclic antidepressants, and injection of medications (usually corticosteroids) into the spine [1,17,18,21,25–28,42–45]. There is some evidence that NSAIDs are effective for chronic LBP [26]. Acetaminophen also can be recommended. While tramadol is of some help [43], there is less evidence for the use of muscle relaxants in chronic LBP [27]. Opioid analgesic therapy for chronic LBP is controversial, but may be of some benefit in a small minority of patients [44]. Tricyclic and tetracyclic antidepressants (but not selective serotonin reuptake inhibitors) have been shown to be of help in patients who have chronic LBP patients but who do not have depression [45].

Injections, usually of corticosteroids, into the spine and usually given into the epidural space are commonly used and may be of some small help, but the evidence is weak [17,21,25,28,42].

Exercise therapy is of some partial help in reducing pain and improving function in patients who have chronic LBP [25,46]. Massage therapy, spinal manipulation, and acupuncture are used for chronic LBP with marginal results [17,21,42]. Physical conditioning programs that include a cognitive behavioral approach are of some benefit as are multidisciplinary programs that include medical, psychologic, and rehabilitative components [42].

Factors that aggravate LBP, such as heavy work, lifting, prolonged sitting or standing, bending or twisting, vibration, monotonous work, job dissatisfaction, and poor relationships with coworkers, should be avoided with the hope that they will lessen current LBP and reduce the risk of worse LBP in the future [21]. Smoking cessation also is recommended [19,21].

The persistent, pernicious nature of chronic LBP in some patients and the frequent occurrence of degenerative changes on imaging studies have led to many different surgical interventions. Various types of spinal fusion are available, and there is evidence that this procedure has been overused in patients who have LBP [47]. Lumbar fusion may be required and helpful for patients who have LBP secondary to spondylolisthesis and spinal instability, but its role for patients who have spondylosis and LBP is controversial. Fusion can be performed from a posterior approach, an anterior approach, or both, usually with some sort of implanted hardware, such as plates and screws or a fusion cage. There are three recent reports of controlled trials of fusion versus conservative treatment [48–52]. The largest study suggested modest improvement in the surgical group, with a 12% to 40% complication rate and a 6% to 17% re-intervention rate [48–50]. Two more recent, smaller studies of instrumented fusion compared with a specific physical therapy program found equal improvement in the two groups [51,52]. A Cochrane review concludes that there is "no scientific evidence about the effectiveness of any form of surgical decompression or fusion for degenerative lumbar spondylosis compared with natural history, placebo, or conservative treatment" [53]. Deyo and colleagues make the "case for restraint" regarding spinal fusion surgery in a recent New England Journal of Medicine article [47].

In October 2004, the United States Food and Drug Administration approved the Charité artificial disk for use in the lumbar spine. This surgery requires an anterior approach with removal of the degenerated disk and placement of the artificial disk. Studies report that the outcomes from placement of an artificial disk are equal to those from lumbar fusion, which is faint praise [54–56]. Longevity of the devices is uncertain, and also there are significant risks with this procedure [56–58]. Total disk replacement in theory preserves motion at the level of the replaced disk, whereas lumbar fusion results in greater motion at the adjacent spinal segments, which could lead to accelerated degenerative changes at these still mobile levels. Artificial cervical and additional artificial lumbar disks currently are being tested in human trials.

After learning about the pros and cons of operative and nonoperative treatments, Patient 5 decided to embark on a physical therapy program, increase his daily dose of ibuprofen, and try to modify his work to lessen the strain placed on his lumbar spine.

Summary

Spine and limb pain related to degenerative, wear-and-tear changes of the disks, joints, and soft tissues of the spine (spondylosis) is exceedingly common. Identical spine and limb pain can be caused by fracture, tumor, or infection. Patients who have a history of significant trauma, signs or symptoms of systemic disease, neurologic impairment, and profound pain require further evaluation, and some may require surgical intervention to decompress the spinal nerves, spinal cord, or cauda equina or to stabilize adjacent spinal segments.

The discovery of red flags in the history or on examination can identify patients who should have imaging and possibly surgical intervention. Neurologic assessment is required to determine which patients could benefit from surgery. The natural history for most acute spondylotic conditions is favorable. Treatment for acute and chronic spine-related pain syndromes is available.

Acknowledgments

The author is deeply appreciative of the superb help provided by Ms. Linda A. Schmidt.

References

[1] Bigos SJ, Bowyer OR, Braen GR, et al. Acute low back problems in adults. Clinical practice guideline and quick reference guide, number 14. Rockville (MD): US Department of Health and Human Services, Public Health Service, Agency for Health Care Policy and Research; December 1994. AHCPR publication number 95-0642 and 95-0643.

[2] Litchy WJ, O'Fallon WM, Kurland LT. Epidemiology of cervical radiculopathy: a population-based study from Rochester, Minnesota, 1976 through 1990. Brain 1994;117:325–35.

[3] Carette S, Fehlings MG. Cervical radiculopathy. N Engl J Med 2005;353:392–9.

[4] Fouyas IP, Statham PFX, Sandercock PAG, et al. Surgery for cervical radiculomyelopathy. Cochrane Database Syst Rev 2005;4:CD001466.

[5] Persson LC, Carlsson CA, Carlsson JY. Long-lasting cervical radicular pain managed with surgery, physiotherapy, or a cervical collar: a prospective, randomized study. Spine 1997;22: 751–8.

[6] Sampath P, Bendebba M, Davis JD, et al. Outcome in patients with cervical radiculopathy: prospective, multicenter study with independent clinical review. Spine 1999;24:591–7.

[7] Levin KH, Covington ED, Devereaux MW, et al. Neck and back pain. Continuum (N Y) 2001;7(1):1–205.

[8] Bartleson JD, O'Duffy JD. Spinal stenosis. In: Koopman WJ, editor. Arthritis and allied conditions. 14th ed. Baltimore: Lippincott Williams & Wilkins; 2001. p. 2042–53.

[9] Lunsford LD, Bissonette DJ, Zorub DS. Anterior surgery for cervical disc disease, part 2: treatment of cervical spondylotic myelopathy in 32 cases. J Neurosurg 1980;53:12–9.

[10] Kumar N, Gross BJ, Ahlskog JE. Copper deficiency myelopathy produces a clinical picture like subacute combine degeneration. Neurology 2004;63:33–9.

[11] Lees F, Turner JWA. Natural history and prognosis of cervical spondylosis. BMJ 1963;2: 1607–10.

[12] Nurick S. The natural history and the results of surgical treatment of the spinal cord disorder associated with cervical spondylosis. Brain 1972;95:101–8.

[13] Ebersold MJ, Pare MC, Quast LM. Surgical treatment for cervical spondylitic myelopathy. J Neurosurg 1995;82:745–51.

[14] Sampath P, Bendebba M, Davis JD, et al. Outcome of patients treated for cervical myelopathy: a prospective, multicenter study with independent clinical review. Spine 2000;25:670–6.

[15] Bednarik J, Kadanka Z, Vohanka S, et al. The value of somatosensory and motor-evoked potentials in predicting and monitoring the effect of therapy in spondylotic cervical myelopathy: prospective randomized study. Spine 1999;24:1593–8.

[16] Kadanka Z, Mares M, Bednanik J, et al. Approaches to spondylotic cervical myelopathy: conservative versus surgical results in a 3-year follow-up study. Spine 2002;27:2205–10.

[17] Deyo RA, Weinstein JN. Low back pain. N Engl J Med 2001;344:363–70.

[18] Bartleson JD. Low back pain and lumbar stenosis. In: Koopman WJ, Boulware DW, Heudebert GR, editors. Clinical primer of rheumatology. Baltimore: Lippincott Williams & Wilkins; 2003. p. 22–42.

[19] Leboeuf-Yde C. Smoking and low back pain: a systematic literature review of 41 journal articles reporting 47 epidemiologic studies. Spine 1999;24:1463–70.

[20] Ahn UM, Ahn NU, Buchowski JM, et al. Cauda equina syndrome secondary to lumbar disc herniation: a meta-analysis of surgical outcomes. Spine 2000;25:1515–22.

[21] Bartleson JD. Low back pain. In: Ringel SP, Swash M, editors. Current treatment options in neurology. Philadelphia: Current Science; 2001. p. 159–68.

[22] Vrooman PCAJ, de Krom MCTFM, Knottnerus JA. Diagnostic value of history and physical examination in patients suspected of sciatica due to disc herniation: a systematic review. Neurology 1999;246:899–906.

[23] Jensen MC, Brant-Zawadzki MN, Obuchowski N, et al. Magnetic resonance imaging of the lumbar spine in people without back pain. N Engl J Med 1994;331:69–73.

[24] Hilde G, Hagen KB, Jamtvedt G, et al. Advice to stay active as a single treatment for low-back pain and sciatica. Cochrane Database Syst Rev 2006;1:CD003632.

[25] van Tulder MW, Koes BW, Bouter LM. Conservative treatment of acute and chronic non-specific low back pain: a systematic review of randomized controlled trials of the most common interventions. Spine 1997;22:2128–56.

[26] van Tulder MW, Scholten RJPM, Koes BW, et al. Nonsteroidal anti-inflammatory drugs for low back pain: a systematic review within the framework of the Cochrane Collaboration Back Review Group. Spine 2000;25:2501–13.

[27] van Tulder MW, Touray T, Furlan AD, et al. Muscle relaxants for non-specific low back pain. Cochrane Database Syst Rev 2005;4:CD004252.

[28] Nelemans PJ, Bie RA, de Vet HCW, et al. Injection therapy for subacute and chronic benign low back pain. Spine 2001;26:501–15.

[29] Gibson JNA, Grant IC, Waddell G. Surgery for lumbar disc prolapse. Cochrane Database Syst Rev 2005;4:CD001350.

[30] Weber H. Lumbar disc herniation: a controlled, prospective study with 10 years of observation. Spine 1983;8:131–40.

[31] Atlas SJ, Deyo RA, Keller RB, et al. The Maine Lumbar Spine Study II. 1-Year outcomes of surgical and nonsurgical management of sciatica. Spine 1996;21:1777–86.

[32] Spivak JM. Degenerative lumbar spinal stenosis. J Bone Joint Surg 1998;80A:1053–66.

[33] Epstein NE, Maldonado VC, Cusick JF. Symptomatic lumbar spinal stenosis. Surg Neurol 1998;103:271–5.

[34] Hall S, Bartleson JD, Onofrio BM, et al. Lumbar spinal stenosis: clinical features, diagnostic procedures, and results of surgical treatment in 68 patients. Ann Intern Med 1985;103:271–5.

[35] Fritz JM, Delitto A, Welch WC, et al. Lumbar spinal stenosis: a review of current concepts in evaluation, management, and outcome measurements. Arch Phys Med Rehabil 1998;79: 700–8.

[36] Atkinson JLD, Miller GM, Krauss WE, et al. Clinical and radiographic features of dural arteriovenous fistula, a treatable cause of myelopathy. Mayo Clin Proc 2001;76:1120–30.

[37] Boden SD, Davis DO, Dina TS, et al. Abnormal magnetic-resonance scans of the lumbar spine in asymptomatic subjects. J Bone Joint Surg [Am] 1990;72:403–8.

[38] Rydevik BL, Cohen DB, Kostuik JP. Spine epidural steroids for patients with lumbar spinal stenosis. Spine 1997;22:2313–7.

[39] Ciol MA, Deyo RA, Howel E, et al. An assessment of surgery for spinal stenosis: time trends, geographic variations, complications, and reoperations. J Am Geriatr Soc 1996;44:285–90.

[40] Deen HG, Zimmerman RS, Lyons MK, et al. Analysis of early failures after lumbar decompressive laminectomy for spinal stenosis. Mayo Clin Proc 1995;70:33–6.

[41] Katz JN, Lipson SJ, Chang LC, et al. Seven-to ten-year outcome of decompressive surgery for degenerative lumbar spinal stenosis. Spine 1996;21:92–8.

[42] Carragee EJ. Persistent low back pain. N Engl J Med 2005;352:1891–8.

[43] Schnitzer TJ, Gray WL, Paster RZ, et al. Efficacy of Tramadol in treatment of chronic low back pain. J Rheumatol 2000;27:772–8.

[44] Bartleson JD. Evidence for and against the use of opioid analgesics for chronic nonmalignant low back pain: a review. Pain Med 2002;3:260–71.

[45] Staiger TO, Gaster B, Sullivan MD, et al. Systematic review of antidepressants in the treatment of chronic low back Pain. Spine 2003;28:2540–5.

[46] Hayden JA, van Tulder MW, Malmivaara AV, et al. Meta-analysis: exercise therapy for nonspecific low back pain. Ann Intern Med 2005;142:765–75.

[47] Deyo RA, Nachemson A, Mirza SK. Spinal-fusion surgery—the case for restraint. N Engl J Med 2004;350:722–6.

[48] Fritzell P, Hagg O, Wessberg P, et al. Lumbar fusion versus nonsurgical treatment for chronic low back pain: a multicenter randomized controlled trial from the Swedish Lumbar Spine Study Group (2001 Volvo Award Winner in Clinical Studies). Spine 2001;26:2521–32.

[49] Fritzell P, Hagg O, Wessberg P, et al. Chronic low back pain and fusion: a comparison of three surgical techniques. Spine 2002;27:1131–41.

[50] Fritzell P, Hagg O, Nordwall A. Complications in lumbar fusion surgery for chronic low back pain: comparison of three surgical techniques used in a prospective randomized study. a report from the Swedish Lumbar Spine Study Group. Eur Spine J 2003;12:178–89.

[51] Ivar Brox J, Sorensen R, Friis A, et al. Randomized clinical trial of lumbar instrumented fusion and cognitive intervention and exercises in patients with chronic low back pain and disc degeneration. Spine 2003;28:1913–21.

[52] Fairbank J, Frost H, Wilson-MacDonald J, et al. Randomised controlled trial to compare surgical stabilisation of the lumbar spine with an intensive rehabilitation programme for patients with chronic low back pain: the MRC Spine Stabilisation Trial. BMJ 2005;330:1233.

[53] Gibson JNA, Waddell G. Surgery for degenerative lumbar spondylosis. Cochrane Database Syst Rev 2005;4:CD001352.

[54] de Kleuver M, Oner FC, Jacobs WC. Total disc replacement for chronic low back pain: background and a systematic review of the literature. Eur Spine J 2003;12:108–16.
[55] German JW, Foley KT. Disc arthroplasty in the management of the painful lumbar motion segment. Spine 2005;30:S60–7.
[56] Blumenthal S, McAfee PC, Guyer RD, et al. A prospective, randomized, multicenter food and drug administration investigational device exemptions study of lumbar total disc replacement with the CHARITE™ artificial disc versus lumbar fusion: part i: evaluation of clinical outcomes. Spine 2005;30:1565–75.
[57] McAfee PC, Fedder IL, Saiedy S, et al. SB Charité disk replacement: report of 60 prospective randomized cases in a us center. J Spinal Disord Tech 2003;16:424–33.
[58] van Ooji A, Oner FC, Verbout AJ. Complications of artificial disk replacement: a report of 27 patients with the SB Charité disc. J Spinal Disord Tech 2003;16:369–83.

ELSEVIER
SAUNDERS

NEUROLOGIC
CLINICS

Neurol Clin 24 (2006) 331–345

Case Studies in Neuro-Ophthalmology for the Neurologist

Andrew G. Lee, MD[a,*], Paul W. Brazis, MD[b]

[a]Departments of Ophthalmology, Neurology, and Neurosurgery,
The University of Iowa Hospitals and Clinics, Iowa City, IA 52242, USA
[b]Departments of Neurology and Ophthalmology, Mayo School of Medicine,
Mayo Clinic, Jacksonville, FL 32224, USA

Neurologists should be familiar with several neuro-ophthalmic conditions that potentially are vision or life threatening. This manuscript concentrates on the following emergent neuro-ophthalmic disorders: (1) temporal (giant cell) arteritis (GCA), (2) intracranial shunt malfunction, (3) idiopathic intracranial hypertension (IIH), (4) pituitary apoplexy, and (5) the pupil-involved third nerve palsy (TNP).

Temporal or giant cell arteritis

Case one

An 85-year-old woman presents with new-onset headache and transient blurred vision in her right eye. An ophthalmologist examines the patient and finds 20/20 visual acuity in both eyes. The remainder of the examination is normal. A carotid Doppler and echocardiogram are normal. An erythrocyte sedimentation rate (ESR) is 25 mm per hour. The patient is referred to a neurologist for the headache and is diagnosed with "migraine with visual aura." The next day the patient loses vision in the right eye to no light perception. She reports scalp tenderness and jaw claudication. There is a right relative afferent pupillary defect and the right optic nerve is swollen (Fig. 1). A C-reactive protein (CRP) is elevated (43 mg/dL; normal, <0.5) and a temporal artery biopsy (TAB) confirms the diagnosis of temporal arteritis. The patient is treated with intravenous (IV) methylprednisolone 1000 mg per day for 5 days followed by oral prednisone at 80 mg

This work was supported in part by an unrestricted grant from Research to Prevent Blindness (New York).

* Corresponding author. Department of Ophthalmology, The University of Iowa Hospitals and Clinics, 200 Hawkins Drive PFP, Iowa City, IA 52242-1091.

E-mail address: andrew-lee@uiowa.edu (A.G. Lee).

0733-8619/06/$ - see front matter © 2006 Elsevier Inc. All rights reserved.
doi:10.1016/j.ncl.2006.01.007

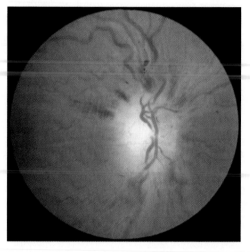

Fig. 1. Fundus photograph shows pallid optic disc edema resulting from arteritic AION.

per day but the vision did not recover. She develops significant steroid-related side effects, including osteoporosis, increased blood sugar, and increased blood pressure and the steroid is tapered over 2 months to a dose of 5 mg of prednisone every other day. At this dosage, the patient loses vision in her left eye to no light perception. A repeat ESR is 100 mm per hour and the CRP now is 26 mg/dL. The prednisone is increased to 100 mg per day but the vision does not recover.

Temporal arteritis, or GCA, is a small- to medium-sized systemic vasculitis that has a predilection for affecting the circulation of the optic nerve and the temporal artery [1–17]. Unfortunately, the constitutional signs and symptoms of GCA can be vague or nonspecific (eg, fatigue, joint pains, fever, and malaise) [4]. Hunder and colleagues reviewed 196 biopsy-proved cases of GCA and 593 other vasculitides [6]. The highest specificity and sensitivity criteria are listed in Box 1. The key to GCA for neurologists is early diagnosis and treatment, before the development of visual loss. The most common errors that neurologists should avoid in the evaluation and management of GCA are listed in Box 2. The diagnosis of GCA should be considered in all elderly patients who have new-onset headache, scalp tenderness, jaw claudication, or visual loss until proved otherwise. Patients who have polymyalgia rheumatica and who present with any of theses symptoms also should be evaluated for GCA.

Treated hydrocephalus and shunt malfunction

Case two

A 26-year-old man has a history of childhood hydrocephalus secondary to aqueductal stenosis. A ventriculoperitoneal (VP) shunt was placed at age 14

Box 1. Criteria for diagnosis of giant cell arteritis

A. Highest sensitivity criteria
1. Age greater than 50 years (mean age 69 years, 90% greater than 60 years)
2. Westergren ESR greater than 50 mm/h (or elevated CRP level)
3. Abnormal TAB

B. Highest specificity clinical criteria
1. Jaw or tongue claudication
2. Visual abnormalities (eg, arteritic ischemic optic neuropathy)
3. Temporal artery abnormalities (eg, decreased pulse, tenderness, or nodules)
4. Neck pain in the elderly (mostly in the occipital and back parts of the neck)

---

and revised at age 16. The patient had decreased vision at the time of the last shunt revision and was noted by ophthalmology to have 20/20 visual acuity, a moderately constricted visual field to 25°, and diffuse optic atrophy in both eyes (Fig. 2). Serial imaging studies have shown stable mild ventriculomegaly with a VP shunt catheter in good position. The patient presents to the emergency department (ED) with new-onset visual loss and mild headache. A repeat CT of the head without contrast shows no change in ventricular size. A shunt series shows the shunt is "connected and intact." The neurosurgery resident on call sees the patient and records in the chart that "the CT scan is stable and that the shunt is functional." The patient is discharged home with follow-up with neurology the next week for the headaches. The next day, however, the vision is worse in both eyes. An ophthalmologist notes 20/50 vision in both eyes, further constriction of the visual field, and diffuse optic atrophy. There is a moderate underaction of elevation of both eyes, light-near dissociation of the pupils, bilateral lid retraction, and convergence-retraction nystagmus in attempted upgaze. A repeat CT scan of the head shows no change. The radiologist reports that the shunt is "functional." The patient's headache and visual loss worsen to counting fingers in both eyes. A second neurosurgeon is called to see the patient. There is slow refilling of the shunt valve clinically. An isotope transport study of the shunt and a shunt pressure measurement confirm shunt malfunction. At the time of shunt revision, the proximal catheter of the shunt is noted to be occluded by choroid plexus. After the shunt revision, however, the vision does not recover.

Any patients who have a history of hydrocephalus treated by an intracranial shunt and who present with a neuro-ophthalmic complaint (eg, visual loss or diplopia) should be considered as having shunt malfunction until proved otherwise. The diagnosis is not difficult in cases with the typical

Box 2. Common errors to avoid in the evaluation of giant cell arteritis

1. Failure to consider occult GCA
   Up to 21% of patients who have biopsy-proved GCA do not
   have any systemic symptoms of GCA (occult GCA) [4,5,9].
   In addition, the lack of visual loss should not dissuade
   neurologists from considering the diagnosis of GCA. Font
   and colleagues report that 65% of patients have two or more
   symptoms of GCA for longer than 3 weeks prior to the visual
   loss [12]. Early identification of patients who have GCA
   without visual loss is key because steroid treatment usually
   does not restore vision but can prevent the onset of visual
   loss.
2. Failure to recognize uncommon neuro-ophthalmic
   manifestations of GCA
   Although the most common cause of visual loss in GCA is
   anterior ischemic optic neuropathy (AION), less common
   causes include nonembolic central retinal artery occlusion,
   cilioretinal artery occlusion, and posterior ischemic optic
   neuropathy [4,5,9]. Transient visual loss (ie, amaurosis
   fugax) and transient diplopia also are potential symptoms of
   GCA. The diplopia in GCA often is transient and variable and,
   typically, is not associated with any deficit on the motility
   examination [4,5,9].
3. Failure to recognize no light perception vision as a sign of GCA
   Severe visual loss worse than counting fingers vision (eg, hand
   motions, light perception, or no light perception) is reported
   in 54% of patients who have AION as a result of GCA
   compared with only 26% of patients who have nonarteritic
   AION. No light perception vision should be considered GCA
   in elderly patients until proved otherwise.
4. Failure to consider GCA in the presence of a normal ESR
   Although the ESR typically is elevated in GCA, a normal ESR
   can occur in 2% to 30% of biopsy-proved cases [4]. In
   addition to the ESR, a CRP may be a more sensitive indicator
   for GCA [5,15] and the combination of the CRP and ESR
   increases the specificity of diagnosis [4,5,9,15].
5. Failure to consider GCA in high-suspicion cases with
   a negative unilateral biopsy
   The pretest likelihood of disease (ie, clinical suspicion for GCA)
   is the best predictor of GCA. If the pretest suspicion for GCA
   is high, then steroid therapy should be initiated regardless of

a normal ESR [4] and regardless of a negative unilateral TAB. If the clinical suspicion remains high after a negative unilateral biopsy, then a contralateral TAB should be considered.

6. Failure to consider GCA as a neuro-ophthalmic emergency
   Untreated GCA blinds affected patients and the visual loss is rapid, often bilateral, and severe. Any patients who have a high suspicion for GCA should be started on empiric steroid therapy and all patients who have visual complaints should be referred to an ophthalmologist. Delay in starting treatment can result in preventable and unnecessary blindness.

7. Failure to start an adequate dose of steroids
   GCA should be treated with high oral dose of prednisone (1.0 mg/kg to 1.5 mg/kg/d; usually 60 to 100 mg/d). Although there is some anecdotal evidence for IV corticosteroids, controlled data is lacking [4,9].

8. Failure to maintain long-term therapy
   Most patients who have GCA require months to years of steroid treatment. An overly aggressive reduction of steroid therapy in GCA may precipitate further visual loss. The dose and duration of steroid treatment should be determined by patient activity of disease symptoms and signs and by the ESR and CRP levels [4,9].

radiographic (ie, ventriculomegaly) or clinical signs and symptoms of shunt malfunction (eg, headache, nausea, vomiting, changes in mental status, and papilledema). Unfortunately, the classic clinical and radiographic findings, including ventricular enlargement, may be absent in patients who have a partially functional or nonfunctional shunt.

Any new or worsening neuro-ophthalmic finding in shunted patients should be considered a sign of shunt failure and visual loss alone can be the presenting or only manifestation. Patients who have severe optic atrophy may not show disc edema because the atrophic nerve fibers cannot manifest swelling. New or increasing findings of the dorsal midbrain syndrome (eg, light-near dissociation of the pupils, convergence-retraction nystagmus, lid retraction, upgaze palsy) or nonlocalizing sixth nerve palsy also should be considered evidence for shunt failure.

It should be emphasized that a "normal" CT scan of the head without recurrent hydrocephalus does not exclude shunt malfunction, because reduced ventricular compliance may not allow ventriculomegaly. A shunt series, a shunt tap, or radionucleotide isotope studies may be necessary to evaluate the shunt fully in patients who have a high clinical suspicion and pretest likelihood for

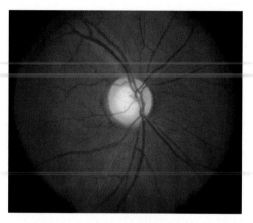

Fig. 2. Fundus photograph shows optic atrophy resulting from prior hydrocephalus with new shunt failure.

shunt failure. Clinicians should consider shunt malfunction in patients who have progressive neuro-ophthalmic findings regardless of the reassurances of radiologists or neurosurgeons based on structural imaging [18–24].

Idiopathic intracranial hypertension

Case three

> A 26-year-old obese woman presents with new-onset headache and blurred vision to the ED. A noncontrast CT scan of the head is normal. A lumbar puncture is performed in the ED to "rule out meningitis or subarachnoid hemorrhage" and showed normal cerebrospinal fluid analysis. No opening pressure is recorded. The patient is discharged from the ED with the diagnosis of "migraine" and scheduled to see a neurologist the following week. The next day, however, the vision deteriorates to counting fingers in each eye. She reports worsening headache, transient visual obscurations, and pulse synchronous tinnitus. An ophthalmologist notes marked visual field constriction in both eyes to 10° and marked papilledema in both eyes (Fig. 3). Cranial MRI with contrast MR venography (MRV) shows only an empty sella. A repeat lumbar puncture shows an opening pressure of 55 cm of water. Oral acetazolamide 1500 mg per day is started. Bilateral optic nerve sheath fenestrations are performed but the vision does not recover.

Papilledema refers to a special form of optic disc edema resulting from increased intracranial pressure. To avoid confusion and to promote clear communication among specialists, the more general descriptive term, optic disc edema, rather than papilledema, should be used for all other causes of optic disc swelling (eg, papillitis, optic neuritis, and AION) [9]. All patients who have bilateral optic disc edema should undergo a blood pressure measurement, because malignant hypertension (grade IV hypertensive

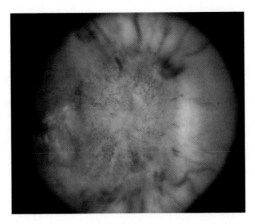

Fig. 3. Fundus photograph shows marked papilledema.

retinopathy) can mimic the clinical presentation of papilledema even in children [24–26]. Hypertension in the setting of papilledema also is a risk factor
for the development of more severe visual loss resulting from superimposed
AION.

Papilledema and increased intracranial pressure may be caused by intracranial neoplasm, venous sinus obstruction, and infectious, inflammatory,
or infiltrative meningeal disease. Although many cases of papilledema are
the result of IIH (ie, pseudotumor cerebri), this is a diagnosis of exclusion
even in obese women [9].The diagnosis of IIH requires the following: (1)
a negative neuroimaging study (preferably contrast-enhanced cranial MR
scan with or without contrast MRV to rule out cerebral venous sinus thrombosis); (2) signs and symptoms related only to increased intracranial pressure
(eg, headache, papilledema, or sixth nerve palsy); (3) a normal cerebrospinal
fluid content; and (4) an elevated opening pressure (more than 200 mm of
water).

Most affected patients (90%) are overweight women and the diagnosis
should be considered with caution in men, elderly patients, and thin patients.
The most common errors in the evaluation and management of IIH are: (1)
failure to order the appropriate neuroimaging study (eg, cranial CT rather
than MRI; lack of MRV, especially in atypical cases; or lack of contrast
MR or MRV); (2) failure to obtain the opening pressure (eg, lumbar puncture
performed in the ED); (3) failure to refer patients who have visual complaints
in a timely manner to ophthalmology for serial visual acuity, visual field testing, and optic disc photography; and (4) failure to refer patients who have
severe visual field loss or acuity loss for an urgent surgical decompression
(eg, optic nerve sheath fenestration or lumboperitoneal shunt) [9].

Neurologists should recognize that IIH potentially is a blinding disorder
and should coordinate the care of these patients with an ophthalmologist or
neuro-ophthalmologist.

Pituitary apoplexy

Case four

A 28-year-old woman presented to the ED on Friday afternoon at 5:00 PM with the "worst headache of her life" and visual loss in both eyes. A non-contrast head CT is interpreted as "normal." A lumbar puncture to "rule out meningitis" or "subarachnoid hemorrhage" is normal. She is given analgesic therapy in the ED and her headache resolves. She is told to make a follow-up appointment with her neurologist for "migraine" the following Monday. The patient has worsening visual loss over the next 2 days, however. An ophthalmologist notes 20/200 acuity in the right eye and 20/20 acuity in the left eye. There is a right relative afferent papillary defect and a bitemporal hemianopsia with a superimposed central scotoma in the right eye. There is a right sixth nerve palsy. Cranial MR scan of the sella shows hyperintense signal intensity consistent with hemorrhage on T1 within a large suprasellar mass arising from the pituitary gland (Fig. 4). There is extension into the suprasellar space with compression of the right optic nerve and chiasm and the lesion involves the right cavernous sinus. The patient is admitted to the hospital and laboratory testing reveals pan-hypopituitarism. She undergoes hormone replacement therapy and an urgent trans-sphenoidal resection of the lesion is performed. The final pathology is infarcted pituitary adenoma with associated hemorrhage. The vision improves to 20/20 in both eyes, but there is residual visual field loss in the right eye and bilateral optic atrophy.

Although generally it is known that a compressive lesion of the optic chiasm produces bitemporal field loss (eg, partial or complete bitemporal hemianopsia with or without paracentral or central field loss), patients who have suprasellar lesions may present with unilateral or bilateral visual loss resulting from compression on one or both optic nerves anteriorly or

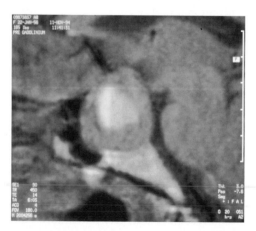

Fig. 4. Sagittal T1-weighted precontrast MRI shows hyperintense signal within a suprasellar mass consistent with pituitary apoplexy.

a homonymous hemianopsia resulting from optic tract compression posteriorly. In addition, if a pituitary lesion expands laterally into the cavernous sinus, patients may present with a pupil abnormality (eg, Horner's syndrome, relative afferent pupillary defect, or TNP-related dilated pupil), ptosis (eg, Horner's syndrome or TNP), or ophthalmoplegia (eg, third, fourth, or sixth nerve palsy). In the acute setting, any of these neuro-ophthalmic presentations may be a sign of hemorrhage or necrosis in a pituitary adenoma (ie, pituitary apoplexy). These patients often report severe headache (eg, "the worst headache of my life"). Acute pituitary insufficiency, especially cortisol deficiency, can be a life-threatening complication of pituitary apoplexy. Appropriate and timely neuroimaging with attention to the sella is critical in making the diagnosis. Urgent surgical intervention may be necessary in patients who have severe visual loss or rapidly expanding lesions.

Pupil-involved isolated third cranial nerve palsy

Case five

> A 55-year-old man presents to the ophthalmologist with new-onset diplopia, ptosis, and headache. The ophthalmologist diagnoses a left TNP. The technician in the eye clinic dilates the pupil and the eye doctor sends the patient to the ED to "rule out aneurysm." A noncontrast CT of the head is negative for subarachnoid hemorrhage. The patient is admitted to the hospital and the neurologist is called the next morning. At morning rounds the patient is examined and noted to have a partial ptosis of the left upper lid; there is underaction of adduction, depression, and elevation of the left eye (Fig. 5) with a 25-prism diopter exotropia and a 10-prism diopter hypotropia in primary position. The pupil is 7 mm in the left eye and 3 mm in the left eye and the left pupil is very sluggishly reactive to light. The remainder of the eye and neurologic examination were normal. Cranial MRI with contrast is normal but a MR angiogram (MRA) suggests a posterior communicating artery aneurysm. Standard catheter angiography reveals an aneurysm at the junction of the left internal carotid artery and the posterior communicating artery. Endovascular interventional therapy with detachable coil is performed with complete obliteration of the aneurysm. Six weeks later, the TNP is resolved completely.

The clinical diagnosis of the classic TNP is straightforward. The typical presentation includes: (1) an ipsilateral ptosis (partial or complete); (2) an ipsilateral exotropia and hypotropia (ie, the eye is "down and out"); and an ipsilateral ophthalmoplegia (eg, adduction, elevation, and depression deficit). Careful measurement of the size and reaction to light for the pupil is critical in the evaluation of the TNP. The simple, but valuable, rule of the pupil states, "pupil involvement in an isolated TNP is due to an aneurysm of posterior communicating artery until proven otherwise" [27–62]. Alternatively, a complete, isolated TNP in vasculopathic patients who have a totally normal pupil (pupil-spared TNP) is unlikely to be an intracranial aneurysm.

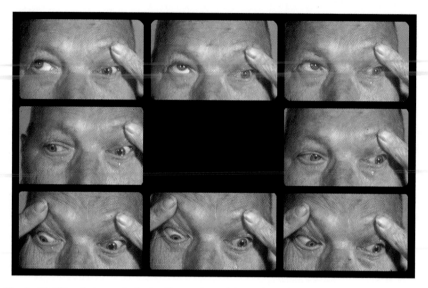

Fig. 5. Motility photographs in the diagnostic positions of gaze demonstrate a partial external dysfunction (more involvement of adduction and elevation and less involvement of depression in the left eye) left third cranial nerve palsy. Note larger pupil in left eye.

Thus, clinicians evaluating patients who have a TNP often are faced with a high stakes decision between a benign (ie, ischemic) etiology and a potentially life-threatening one (ie, aneurysm).

Patients who have an isolated TNP can be divided into those who have complete or incomplete external (eg, lid and motility) and internal (ie, the pupil) dysfunction. For example, a complete external dysfunction TNP involves all of the somatic branches of the third nerve and there is total or almost total paralysis of these involved muscles. A partial external dysfunction TNP might not involve all of the somatic branches of the third nerve (eg, superior divisional palsy) or might produce an incomplete paralysis of these muscles (eg, minimal ptosis, mild adduction, or depression deficit, but a marked elevation deficit or any other similar combination of partial external dysfunction).

The complete external dysfunction TNP may be associated with complete internal dysfunction (ie, a fixed and dilated pupil), partial internal dysfunction (ie, partial pupil involvement or partial pupil sparing), or no internal dysfunction (ie, pupil sparing). True pupil sparing should apply only to the TNP with complete external dysfunction and not to incomplete external dysfunction TNP (eg, divisional palsies). Thus, clinicians should be cautious when interpreting the significance of lack of internal dysfunction (ie, pupil sparing) in the setting of partial external dysfunction.

Patients who have an isolated, complete external dysfunction but normal internal function (ie, pupil-spared) TNP should be evaluated for underlying vasculopathic risk factors (hypertension, diabetes, older age, and so forth)

even in the absence of any history of these ischemic etiologies. An acute, isolated TNP with complete external dysfunction but no internal dysfunction
(ie, pupil spared) may be observed for improvement over time (usually
6 to 8 weeks) and presumed ischemic in patients who are vasculopathic.
The pupil examination should be repeated within the next few days to insure
that internal dysfunction (ie, pupil involvement) does not occur. Patients
who have no known vasculopathic risk factors, even with a complete external dysfunction and a normal pupil, probably should undergo neuroimaging
(preferably MRI and MRA of the head). Evaluation for myasthenia gravis
also should be performed in any pupil-spared, nonproptotic, nonpainful,
isolated ocular motor deficit, including the pupil-spared TNP.

Patients who have a partial external dysfunction TNP may seem to spare
the pupil but the rule of the pupil and of pupil sparing should be applied with
caution in this setting. The pupil may seem to be spared in a TNP with partial external dysfunction (eg, superior division TNP) because that portion of
the third nerve that carries the pupil fibers may not be involved significantly.
Although an aneurysm causing a TNP impairs the pupil in 96% of cases, in
the remaining 4% of cases, the pupil presumably was not involved, because
the TNP had only partial external dysfunction [63,64]. There are several cases
of supposed pupil-sparing TNP resulting from aneurysm with partial external dysfunction TNP [28,30–33,37,39–45,47–50,58–62]. The rule of the pupil
in terms of the clinical significance of pupil sparing should be used with caution in partial external dysfunction TNP and probably should be reserved for
complete external dysfunction TNP.

The partial external dysfunction TNP with normal internal function
probably still requires a cranial MR scan with contrast to rule out a mass
lesion and an MRA. If the MR and MRA are normal, cerebral angiography
(the gold standard) still may be necessary depending on the clinical scenario
and the pretest likelihood for aneurysm [36,51].

Likewise, patients who have partial internal dysfunction (ie, relative pupil
sparing) can present with either a small degree of anisocoria or a diminished
but present light reflex. The partial internal dysfunction TNP with either
partial or complete external dysfunction also should have MRI and MRA
or CT angiography (CTA). Cullom and coworkers prospectively studied
10 patients who had partial internal dysfunction (ie, relative pupillary sparing) TNP and none of the patients demonstrated aneurysm [32]. Although
Cullom and coworkers suggest that the prevalence of aneurysm in this population was low, the sample size was too small to make an evidence-based
recommendation and internal carotid artery, posterior communicating artery, and basilar artery aneurysms are reported in isolated TNP with so-
called "relative pupillary sparing" [28,31,34,37,41,43].

Patients who have no external dysfunction but partial or complete internal dysfunction do not have a TNP and are more likely to harbor a pupil
abnormality (eg, iris sphincter tear or post-traumatic or post-surgical anisocoria), damage to the ciliary ganglion (eg, tonic pupil), or pharmacologic

Table 1
Risk of intracranial aneurysm and recommended evaluation based on degree of internal (ie, pupil) and external dysfunction of the neurologically isolated third nerve palsy

Degree of internal dysfunction	Complete external dysfunction	Partial external dysfunction	No external dysfunction
Complete internal dysfunction (ie, pupil involved)	• Highest risk • MRI with MRA (CTA) • Catheter angiography probably still required	• Highest risk • MRI with MRA (CTA) • Catheter angiography probably still required	Not likely to be a TNP (eg, traumatic, Adie's pupil, pharmacologic)
Partial internal dysfunction (ie, relative pupil sparing)	• Uncertain, but probably low risk • MRI with MRA (CTA) • Consider catheter angiography[a]	• Uncertain, but probably low risk • MRI with MRA (CTA) • Consider catheter angiography[a]	Not likely to be a TNP (eg, traumatic, Adie's pupil, pharmacologic)
No internal dysfunction (normal pupil)	• Low risk of aneurysm in vasculopathic patient' observe • MRI with MRA (CTA) if nonvasculopathic or unresolved	• Uncertain risk • MRI with MRA (CTA) • Consider catheter angiography[a]	Not applicable

[a] Depends on the reliability of local neuroimaging (eg, MRI, MRA, CTA) and the pretest likelihood of aneurysm based on clinical suspicion. If the pretest likelihood is low or if the risk of catheter angiography is unreasonably high (eg, elderly, high risk of renal failure, risk of stroke), then an MRI and MRA (or CTA) may be a reasonable test. Thus, individual patients still may require catheter angiography even if the MRI with MRA (CTA) is negative, depending on the pretest likelihood for aneurysm.

From Lee AG. Third cranial nerve palsy. Available at: http://www.ophthalmic.hyperguides. com. Accessed November 2004. Courtesy of Ophthalmic Hyperguides; with permission.

dilation. Patients who have a dilated pupil alone without ptosis or motility deficit generally do not require imaging and should be evaluated for alternative etiologies to TNP for their anisocoria.

Although conventional catheter arteriography remains the gold standard for the diagnosis of cerebral aneurysms, newer and relatively noninvasive angiography techniques, including MRA and CTA, are approaching the sensitivity and specificity of catheter angiograms. The techniques continue to evolve and a properly performed and interpreted MRI with MRA (or CTA) has a sensitivity of 98% for the detection of an aneurysm producing a TNP [63,64]. Table 1 lists proposed imaging guidelines for TNP.

Summary

In summary, neurologists should be aware of emergent neuro-ophthalmic conditions: (1) temporal arteritis (GCA), (2) IIH, (3) intracranial shunt malfunction, (4) pituitary apoplexy, and (5) pupil-involved TNP. Earlier recognition and treatment of these disorders makes a difference in final outcome. Appropriate evaluation and management may be vision or life saving.

References

[1] Cullen FP. Occult temporal arteritis. A common cause of blindness in old age. Br J Ophthalmol 1967;51:513–25.
[2] Fernandez-Herlihy L. Temporal arteritis: clinical aids to diagnosis. J Rheumatol 1988;15: 1797–801.
[3] Goodman BW Jr. Temporal arteritis. Am J Med 1979;67:839–52.
[4] Lee AG, Brazis PW. Temporal arteritis: a clinical approach. J Am Geriatr Soc 1999;47: 1364–70.
[5] Hayreh SS, Podhajsky PA, Raman R, et al. Giant cell arteritis: validity and reliability of various diagnostic criteria. Am J Ophthalmol 1997;123:285–96.
[6] Hunder GG, Bloch DA, Michel BA, et al. The American College of Rheumatology 1990 criteria for the classification of giant cell arteritis. Arthritis Rheum 1990;33:1122–8.
[7] Mizen TR. Giant cell arteritis: diagnostic and therapeutic considerations. Ophthalmol Clin North Am 1991;4:547–56.
[8] Rosenfeld SI, Kosmorsky GS, Klingele TG, et al. Treatment of temporal arteritis with ocular involvement. Am J Med 1986;80:143–5.
[9] Lee AG, Brazis PW. Clinical pathways in neuro-ophthalmology: an evidence-based approach. New York: Thieme; 1998. p. 67–91.
[10] Vilaseca J, Gonzalez A, Cid MC, et al. Clinical usefulness of temporal artery biopsy. Ann Rheum Dis 1987;46:282–5.
[11] Chmelewski WL, McKnight KM, Agudelo CA, et al. Presenting features and outcome in patients undergoing temporal artery biopsy: a review of 98 patients. Arch Intern Med 1992;152:1690–5.
[12] Font C, Ced MC, Coll-Vinent B, et al. Clinical features in patients with permanent visual loss due to biopsy-proven giant cell arteritis. Br J Ophthalmol 1997;36:251–4.
[13] Sox HC, Liang MH. The erythrocyte sedimentation rate: guidelines for rational use. Ann Intern Med 1986;104:515.
[14] Miller A, Green M. Simple rule for calculating normal erythrocyte sedimentation rate. BMJ 1983;286:266.
[15] Eshaghian J, Goeken JA. C-reactive protein in giant cell (cranial, temporal) arteritis. Ophthalmol 1980;87:1160–6.
[16] Cornblath WT, Eggenberger E. Progressive visual loss from giant cell arteritis despite high-dose intravenous methylprednisolone. Ophthalmology 1997;104:854–8.
[17] Hayreh SS. Anterior ischaemic optic neuropathy. Differentiation of arteritis from nonarteritic type and its management. Eye 1990;4:25.
[18] Lee AG. Visual loss as the manifesting symptom of ventriculoperitoneal shunt malfunction. Am J Ophthalmol 1996;122:127–9.
[19] Chou SY, Digre KB. Neuro-ophthalmic complications of raised intracranial pressure, hydrocephalus, and shunt malfunction. Neurosurg Clin North Am 1999;10:587–608.
[20] Corbett JJ. Neuro-ophthalmologic complications of hydrocephalus and shunting procedures. Semin Neurol 1986;6:111–23.
[21] Engel M, Carmel PW, Chutorian AM. Increased intraventricular pressure without ventriculomegaly in children with shunts: "normal volume" hydrocephalus. Neurosurgery 1979;5: 549–52.
[22] Newman NJ. Bilateral visual loss and disc edema in a 15-year-old girl. Surv Ophthalmol 1994;38:365–70.
[23] Arroyo HA, Jan JE, McCormick AQ, et al. Permanent visual loss after shunt malfunction. Neurology 1985;35:25–9.

[24] Trobe JD. Neuro-ophthalmic diagnoses you don't want to miss. Focal Points 1999;9:1–14.

[25] Lip GY, Beevers M, Dodson PM, et al. Severe hypertension with lone bilateral papilloedema: a variant of malignant hypertension. Blood Press 1999;4:339–42.

[26] Hayreh SS, Servais GE, Virdi PS. Fundus lesions in malignant hypertension. V Hypertensive optic neuropathy. Ophthalmology 1986;93:74–87.

[27] Trobe JD. Isolated pupil-sparing third nerve palsy. Ophthalmology 1985;92:58–61.

[28] Lustbader JM, Miller NR. Painless, pupil-sparing, but otherwise complete oculomotor paresis caused by basilar artery aneurysm. Arch Ophthalmol 1988;106:583–4.

[29] Jacobson DM. Pupil involvement in patients with diabetes-associated oculomotor nerve palsy. Arch Ophthalmol 1998;116:723–7.

[30] Naudea SE, Trobe JD. Pupil sparing in oculomotor palsy: a brief review. Ann Neurol 1983; 13:143–8.

[31] Kissel JT, Burde RM, Klingele TG, et al. Pupil-sparing oculomotor palsies with internal carotid-posterior communicating artery aneurysms. Ann Neurol 1983;15:149–54.

[32] Cullom ME, Savino PJ, Sergott RC, et al. Relative pupillary sparing third nerve palsies. To angiogram or not? J Neuroophthalmol 1995;15:136–41.

[33] Bartleson JD, Trautmann JC, Sundt TM. Minimal oculomotor nerve paresis secondary to unruptured intracranial aneurysm. Arch Neurol 1986;43:1015–20.

[34] Kasoff I, Kelly DL. Pupillary sparing oculomotor palsies with internal carotid-posterior communicating artery aneurysms. J Neurosurg 1975;42:713–7.

[35] Goldstein JE, Cogan DG. Diabetic ophthalmoplegia with special reference to the pupil. Arch Ophthalmol 1960;64:592–600.

[36] Kaufman DI. Recent advances in neuro-imaging and the impact on neuro-ophthalmology. Curr Opin Ophthalmol 1994;5:52–62.

[37] Guy JR, Day AL. Intracranial aneurysms with superior division paresis of the oculomotor nerve. Ophthalmology 1989;96:1071–6.

[38] Hopf HC, Gutmann L. Diabetic third nerve palsy: evidence for a mesencephalic lesion. Neurol 1990;40:1041–5.

[39] Crompton JL, Moore CE. Painful third nerve palsy: how not to miss an intracranial aneurysm. Aust J Ophthalmol 1981;9:113–5.

[40] DiMario FJJ, Rorke LB. Transient oculomotor nerve paresis in congenital distal basilar artery aneurysm. Pediatr Neurol 1992;8:303–6.

[41] Feder R, Camp WA. Superior branch palsy of oculomotor nerve and pupillary constriction caused by intracranial carotid artery aneurysm. Ann Neurol 1979;5:493–5.

[42] Gale AN, Crockard HA. Transient unilateral mydriasis with basilar aneurysm. J Neurol Neurosurg Psychiatry 1982;45:565–6.

[43] Good EF. Ptosis as the sole manifestation of compression of the oculomotor nerve by an aneurysm of the posterior communicating artery. J Clin Neuroophthalmol 1990;10:59–61.

[44] Greenspan BN, Reeves AG. Transient partial oculomotor nerve paresis with posterior communicating aneurysm — a case report. J Clin Neuroophthalmol 1990;10:56–8.

[45] Griffiths PD, Gholkar A, Sengupta RP. Oculomotor nerve palsy due to thrombosis of a posterior communicating artery aneurysm following diagnostic angiography. Neuroradiol 1994; 36:614–5.

[46] McFadzean RM, Teasdale EM. Computerized tomography angiography in isolated third nerve palsies. J Neurosurg 1998;88:679–84.

[47] Payne JW, Adamkiewicz J Jr. Unilateral internal ophthalmoplegia with intracranial aneurysm. Report of a case. Am J Ophthalmol 1969;68:349–52.

[48] Ranganadham P, Dinakar I, Mohandas S, et al. A rare presentation of posterior communicating artery aneurysm. Clin Neurol Neurosurg 1992;94:225–7.

[49] Soni SR. Aneurysms of the posterior communicating artery and oculomotor nerve paresis. J Neurol Neurosurg Psychiatry 1974;37:1803–8.

[50] Soria E, Camell H, Dang H. Pupil-sparing oculomotor palsy caused by fusiform arteriosclerotic aneurysm of the basilar artery—a case report. Angiology 1989;40:921–7.

[51] Teasdale E, Stratham P, Straiton J, et al. Non-invasive radiological investigation for oculo-motor palsy. J Neurol Neurosurg Psychiatry 1990;53:549–53.

[52] Walter KA, Newman NJ, Lessell S. Oculomotor palsy from minor head trauma: initial sign of intracranial aneurysm. Neurology 1994;44:148–50.

[53] Wolin MJ, Saunders RA. Aneurysmal oculomotor nerve palsy in an 11-year-old boy. J Clin Neuroophthalmol 1992;12:178–80.

[54] Asbury AK, Aldridge H, Hersberg R, et al. Oculomotor palsy in diabetes mellitus: a clinico-pathological study. Brain 1970;93:555–66.

[55] Berlit P. Isolated and combined pareses of cranial nerves III, IV, and VI. A retrospective study of 412 patients. J Neurol Sci 1991;103:10–5.

[56] Bortolami R, D'Alessandro R, Manni E. The origin of pain in 'ischemic-diabetic' third-nerve palsy. Arch Neurol 1993;50:795.

[57] Dreyfus PM, Hakim S, Adams RD. Diabetic ophthalmoplegia: report of case with post-mortem study and comments on vascular supply of human oculomotor nerve. Arch Neurol Psychiatry 1975;77:337–49.

[58] Cogan DG, Mount HTJ. Intracranial aneurysms causing ophthalmoplegia. Arch Ophthal-mol 1963;70:757–71.

[59] Hepler RS, Cantu RC. Aneurysms and third nerve palsies. Arch Ophthalmol 1967;77:604–8.

[60] O'Connor PS, Tredici TJ, Green RP. Pupil-sparing third nerve palsies caused by aneurysms. Am J Ophthalmol 1983;95:395–7.

[61] Zingale A, Albanese V, Giuffrida A, et al. Painful ophthalmoplegia syndrome (spheno-cavernous syndrome) caused by a ruptured posterior communicating artery aneurysm. A brief report. J Neurosurg Sci 1997;41:299–301.

[62] Zimmer DV. Oculomotor nerve palsy from posterior communicating artery aneurysm. J LA State Med Soc 1991;143:22–5.

[63] Jacobson DM, Trobe JD. The emerging role of magnetic resonance angiography in the man-agement of patients with third cranial nerve palsy. Am J Ophthalmol 1999;28:94–6.

[64] Trobe JD. Managing oculomotor nerve palsy. Arch Ophthalmol 1998;116:798.

ELSEVIER
SAUNDERS

NEUROLOGIC
CLINICS

Neurol Clin 24 (2006) 347–362

Case Studies of Uncommon Headaches

Randolph W. Evans, MD[a,b,c]

[a]Department of Neurology and Neuroscience, Weill Medical College of Cornell University,
New York, NY, USA
[b]Department of Neurology, The Methodist Hospital, Houston, TX, USA
[c]Department of Neurology, Baylor College of Medicine, Houston, TX, USA

The following nine cases present uncommon but fascinating primary and secondary headache disorders. If you are not already familiar with or have not seen these disorders, you will be prepared when someone presents or a colleague asks you about an unusual case.

Case 1. Noises in the night

A 43-year-old woman was seen with a 5-month history of a noise in her head. On an almost nightly basis, as she was falling asleep, she would hear a loud noise like "electrical current running" lasting a second. Sometimes her whole body would shake for a second afterwards. Very occasionally, she would have an associated flash of light. Frequently, a second episode of the loud noise occurred shortly after the first. She then could fall asleep without any problem.

Her medical history was positive only for hypertension controlled with medication. Neurologic examination was normal. Diagnostic testing was not performed [1].

Questions

What is the diagnosis? Which type of headaches can awaken patients from sleep?

Discussion

These episodes are characteristic of exploding head syndrome, a disorder named by Pearce in 1988 [2]. Episodes of exploding head syndrome, which occur on falling asleep or, less often, on awakening, awaken people from

---

1200 Binz #1370, Houston, TX 77004.
E-mail address: rwevans@pol.net

0733-8619/06/$ - see front matter © 2006 Elsevier Inc. All rights reserved.
doi:10.1016/j.ncl.2006.01.006

sleep with a sensation of a loud bang in the head, like an explosion. Ten percent of cases are associated with the perception of a flash of light. Five percent of patients report a curious sensation as if they had stopped breathing and had to make a deliberate effort to breathe again. The episodes have a variable frequency and onset at any age, although the most common is middle age and older. The episodes take place in healthy individuals during any stage of sleep without evidence of epileptogenic discharges. The basis of this syndrome may be a delay in the reduction of activity in selected areas of the brainstem reticular formation as the patient passes from wakefulness to sleep. Symptoms typically resolve with time and with reassurance that the disorder is benign.

Secondary causes of nocturnal headaches include drug withdrawal, temporal arteritis, sleep apnea, nocturnal hypertension-headache syndrome, oxygen desaturation, pheochromocytomas, primary and secondary neoplasms, communicating hydrocephalus, subdural hematomas, subacute angle-closure glaucoma, and vascular lesions [3]. Migraine, cluster, hypnic, and chronic paroxysmal hemicrania are primary headaches that can cause awakening from sleep. Migraine typically has associated symptoms and uncommonly occurs only during sleep. Cluster headaches have autonomic symptoms and may occur during the day and during sleep. Chronic paroxysmal hemicrania occurs during the day and at night, lasts for less than 30 minutes, and occurs 10 to 30 times a day.

Case 2. Headache causing awakening from sleep

A 56-year-old man who had a history of well-controlled hypertension and episodic tension-type headache was awoken from sleep 3 nights per month for the past 2 years between 1:00 AM and 2:30 AM with a moderately severe bifrontal pressing headache, which persisted for 1 to 2 hours untreated and 10 minutes if treated with a caffeine-containing over-the-counter analgesic [4].

Questions

What is the diagnosis? Which other treatments might be effective?

Discussion

Hypnic headache is a rare disorder, first reported by Raskin in 1988 [5], that occurs more often in the elderly (but with a range of 36 to 83 years of age and a single case of a 9 year old [6]) with a female predominance [7]. The headaches occur only during sleep and awaken the sufferer at a consistent time. Nausea is infrequent, and autonomic symptoms are rare. The headaches can be unilateral or bilateral, throbbing or nonthrobbing, and mild to severe in intensity. During the headaches, patients typically prefer to sit up or stand, as lying supine may intensify the pain. The headaches can last 15 minutes to 3 hours and can occur frequently, as often as nightly, for many years. Spontaneous resolution is uncommon. There are two case reports of secondary hypnic headache: one patient who had obstructive sleep apnea with resolution of headaches with use of continuous positive airway pressure [8] and a second who had a posterior fossa meningioma with resolution of headaches after removal [9].

Medications reported as effective include caffeine (one or two cups of caffeinated coffee or a 40- to 60-mg caffeine tablet before bedtime), lithium carbonate (300 mg at bedtime), indomethacin, atenolol, melatonin, cyclobenzaprine, verapamil, pizotifen, gabapentin, clonidine, acetylsalicyclic acid, acetaminophen, ergotamine derivatives, acetazolamide, prednisone, and flunarizine (not available in the United States). The diagnosis is one of exclusion.

Case 3. Numb tongue

This is a 15-year-old boy who had a history of migraines since approximately age 4. The migraines occur approximately once every 6 months and are described as a severe bifrontal throbbing associated with nausea, light and noise sensitivity, and sometimes vomiting but no aura. The headaches last approximately a half day, and he often goes to bed during the attack. Acetaminophen is of mild help.

For the past 6 months, he has developed a new type of headache, occurring approximately once every 2 weeks. These headaches are triggered by activity, such as throwing a football hard, hitting an overhead ball in tennis, or chasing his dog around in a circle, but not by weightlifting or straining with a bowel movement. He describes a sharp pain in the mid nuchal-occipital region associated with numbness of the left side of the tongue, all lasting approximately 20 seconds.

Medical history is negative except for congenital bilateral hearing loss. Family history is remarkable for migraines in his father and congenital hearing loss. Neurologic examination is normal, except for profound hearing loss bilaterally. MRI scan of the brain shows a large retrocerebellar arachnoid cyst without hydrocephalus. The cerebellar tonsils are above the foramen magnum [10].

Question

What is the cause of the transient episodes of nuchal-occipital pain and numbness of the left side of the tongue?

Discussion

This teenager has neck-tongue syndrome first described by Lance and Anthony in 1980 [11]. The arachnoid cyst is an incidental finding. Neck-tongue syndrome is an uncommon disorder characterized by acute unilateral occipital pain and numbness of the ipsilateral tongue lasting seconds to 1 minute and precipitated by sudden movement, usually rotation, of the head. The symptoms are the result of transient subluxation of the atlantoaxial joint that stretches the joint capsule and the C2 ventral ramus, which contains proprioceptive fibers from the tongue originating from the lingual nerve to the hypoglossal nerve to the C2 root (Fig. 1). Although neck-tongue syndrome can occur without obvious abnormalities, associated disorders include degenerative spondylosis, ankylosing spondylitis, psoriatic arthritis, and genetically determined laxity of ligaments of joint capsules. A benign, familial form of neck-tongue syndrome is described without anatomic abnormality, which resolves spontaneously during adolescence [12].

Case 4. I feel really big, no make that really small

A 31-year-old woman has a 10-year history of mild headaches occurring approximately once in a month. For the past 6 months, the headaches have increased in frequency and severity, occurring 5 days per week, and are described as a pressure around her eyes with nausea and light sensitivity typically of moderate intensity but severe once a week lasting many hours. There was no aura. There is no family history of migraine. Neurologic examination was normal. A MRI scan of the brain was normal. She was started on topiramate (25 mg daily) to be increased by 25 mg per week to 100 mg per day.

When seen at follow-up 1 month later, the headaches were mild and had decreased to 1 or 2 per week. She reported, however, having five episodes during the prior 3 weeks lasting 2 to 3 minutes and followed by a mild pressure headache behind her eyes lasting 30 to 45 minutes without medication. With three of the episodes, she felt like her entire body was

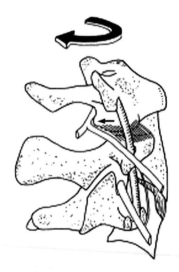

Fig. 1. A lateral view of a right atlantoaxial joint in which the atlas has rotated to the right. (*From* Evans RW, Lance JW. Transient headache with numbness of half of the tongue. Headache 2000;40:692–3; with permission.)

too big and everything else was too small. With two of the episodes, she had a feeling that her entire body was too small and everything else too big. During the episodes, however, everything actually looked normal and she was aware her abnormal feeling was not real. An EEG was normal.

At follow-up 5 weeks later, she reported eight episodes all lasting approximately 5 to 10 minutes. During four of the episodes she reported feeling too small and with two, too big. With two episodes, she felt too big for approximately 5 minutes and then too small for approximately 5 minutes. All of the episodes were followed by the mild headache lasting approximately 1 hour [13].

Questions

What is the diagnosis? What is the derivation of the name of this disorder?

Discussion

"Alice in Wonderland" syndrome is a rare migraine aura where patients experience distortion in body image characterized by enlargement, diminution, or distortion of part of or the whole body, which they know is not real. The syndrome can occur at any age but is more common in children. The cause may be migrainous ischemia of the nondominant posterior parietal lobule. Although most common with migraine, it also is reported after viral encephalitis (especially after Epstein-Barr virus) and as an epileptic phenomenon.

Although previously not reported as a side effect of medication use, case four's "Alice in Wonderland" syndrome may be associated with topiramate use [14]. Her visual symptoms started 1 week after starting topiramate and resolved 1 month after stopping topiramate (2.5 months after initiation). After follow up 2 years and 9 months later, she had no further episodes. This association seems plausible with my recent report [14] of two migraneurs with reversible palinpopsia associated with topiramate use. Both sufferers had resolution of the palinposia on discontinuation of topiramate and the same visual symptoms again when topiramate was restarted.

Lippman describes seven migraineurs who had unusual distortions of body image in 1952 [15]. The descriptions of four patients are illustrative: "Occasionally the patient has an attack where she feels small, about 1 ft high." Another patient had the sensation of "her left ear ballooning out six inches or more." A third patient described his sensations: "the body is as if someone had drawn a vertical line separating the two halves. The right half seems to be twice the size of the left half." And a fourth noted, "I feel that my body is growing larger and larger until it seems to occupy the whole room."

In 1955, Todd gave the syndrome its name [16] from the book, *Alice's Adventures in Wonderland*, published in England in 1864 by Charles

Lutwidge Dodgson under the pseudonym of Lewis Carroll (the Latinization of Lutwidge Charles). Dodgson was a Professor of Mathematics at Oxford University and a migraineur. There is speculation that he might have had the syndrome [17,18].

In the first chapter of the book, Alice jumps down a rabbit hole and lands in a hallway where she finds a bottle, which she drinks from, causing her to shrink: "'I must be shutting up like a telescope.' And so it was indeed: she was now only 10 in high …'" Later, she eats a piece of cake that makes her grow (Fig. 2): "'Curiouser and couriouser!' cried Alice…; 'now I'm opening out like the largest telescope that ever was! Good-bye, feet!' (for when she looked down at her feet, they seemed to be almost out of sight, they were getting so far off.)" Neurologic topics related to another character introduced in the first chapter, the White Rabbit, are beyond the scope of this discussion.

Neuroimaging studies in migraineurs with the syndrome are normal. Patients who have frequent Alice in Wonderland auras may benefit from migraine preventive medications.

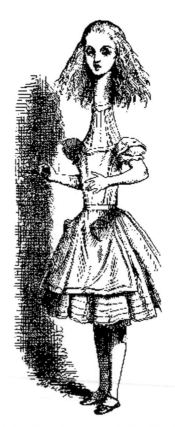

Fig. 2. Alice stretched tall. (Illustration by Sir John Tenniel, 1865).

Other rare visual hallucinations, distortions, and illusions that are reported in migraine include the following: zoopsia (visual hallucinations containing complex objects, such as people and animals); achromatopsia (no perception of color); prosopagnosia (inability to recognize faces); visual agnosia (inability to recognize objects); akinetopsia (loss of ability to perceive visual motion); metamorphopsia (distortion of the shapes of objects); micropsia (objects appear too small); macropsia (objects appear too small); teleopsia (objects seem too far away); lilliputianism (people appear too small); multiple images; persistent positive visual phenomena (diffuse small particles, such as TV static or dots, in the entire visual field lasting months to years); palinopsia (the persistence or recurrence of visual images after the exciting stimulus object isn removed); cerebral polyopia (the perception of multiple images); and tilted and upside-down vision [19].

Case 5. My scalp hurts

A 45-year-old woman presents with a 3-month history of a scalp pain. She describes a burning, stinging, itching, and sore pain of the midposterior frontal and anterior parietal scalp in an elliptic distribution extending across both sides with a diameter of approximately 5 cm. The pain is present intermittently daily, lasting hours at a time with an intensity of 5/10. At times, the area is sensitive when she brushes her hair. Ibuprofen may reduce the discomfort. She has seen two dermatologists who found normal skin examinations. There is no history of migraine or other headaches. There is a medical history of hypertension. Neurologic examination was normal with no abnormality of scalp sensation.

MRI of the brain was normal. Blood work was normal, including the following: erythrocyte sedimentation rate, 12 mm per hour; rheumatoid factor, 11 IU/mL; antinuclear antibody (ANA) screen, negative; serum protein electrophoresis, normal; serum immunofixation, showing no monoclonal immunoglobin; Sjögren's antibodies A and B, negative; vitamin B_{12} level, 743 pg/mL; and thyrotropin, 1.5. The patient was placed on gabapentin (100 mg by mouth three times a day), which she took as needed with a reduction in the level of pain to a 2/10 [20].

Question

What is the diagnosis?

Discussion

After seeing this patient, I had no idea of the diagnosis. Several hours later, I was reading an article by Pareja and colleagues [21] during lunch and immediately recognized her problem. Nummular headache (a coin-shaped cephalalgia) is a rare, chronic, mild to moderate, pressure-like pain in a rounded or elliptic scalp area (most often the parietal region, in particular its most convex portion, although any region of the head may be affected) of approximately 1 to 6 cm in diameter first described by Pareja and colleagues in 2002 [22,23]. The location usually is single and unilateral, not changing in size or shape with time, but it can be midline and bilateral as in this case [24]. Typically, the pain is continuous and persists for days to months with exacerbations described as lancinating pains lasting for several seconds or minutes up to a few hours. The affected area may show a variable combination of hypoesthesia, dysesthesia, paresthesia, or tenderness. Spontaneous remissions may occur but the pain usually recurs.

Diagnostic testing, including CT, MRI of the brain, and blood work, is normal. Mild cases typically require no treatment. Patients who have more intense pain might benefit from naproxen or gabapentin. Although the cause is not known, the disorder is benign and might be the result of a localized terminal branch neuralgia of a pericranial nerve.

Case 6. My ear is red, hot, and burning

A 54-year-old white woman was seen who had a 10-year history of episodes of a burning sensation of the left ear. The episodes are preceded by nausea and a hot feeling for approximately 15 seconds and then the left ear becomes visibly red for an average of approximately 1 hour, with a range of approximately 30 minutes to 2 hours. Approximately once every 2 years, she had a flurry of episodes occurring over approximately a 1-month period during which she averaged approximately five episodes, with a range of 1 to 6.

There also was an 18-year history of migraine without aura occurring approximately once a year. At the age of 36, she developed left-sided pulsatile tinnitus. A cerebral arteriogram revealed a proximal left internal carotid artery occlusion of uncertain cause after extensive testing. MRI scan at age 45 was normal. Neurologic examination was normal. A carotid ultrasound study demonstrated complete occlusion of the left internal carotid artery and a normal right [25].

Question

What is the diagnosis?

Discussion

Lance first described the red ear syndrome in 1995 [26] and also proposes the term, auriculoautonomic cephalgia. The disorder is characterized by episodic burning pain, usually in one ear lobe, associated with flushing or reddening of the ear with a duration of 5 minutes to 3 hours in children and adults [27]. In individuals, one ear, alternating ears, or occasionally both ears can be involved in attacks that can occur rarely or up to 4 per day. The redness can occur without pain. Frequent episodes might be reduced with preventive use of gabapentin.

The syndrome can be idiopathic or occur in association with migraine (during or between headache episodes) [27,28], thalamic syndrome, atypical glossopharyngeal and trigeminal neuralgia, upper cervical spine pathology (cervical arachnoiditis, cervical spondylosis, traction injury, Chiari malformation, or herpes zoster of the upper cervical roots), and dysfunction of the temporomandibular joint [29–31]. Lance postulates that the cause might be an antidromic discharge of nerve impulses in the third cervical root and greater auricular nerve in response to some local pain-producing lesion in the upper neck or trigeminal areas of innervation. In this case, the red ear syndrome probably is associated with migraine and the carotid occlusion an incidental finding.

Case 7. My mouth is burning

A 49-year-old woman was referred by her primary care physician with a 1.5-year history of daily constant burning or numbness of the entirety of her tongue and the back of her throat. She also complains that the inside of her mouth is sensitive. She has had a dry mouth for the past year. She had seen an ear, nose, and throat physician, gastroenterologist, and dentist. Artificial saliva has not been helpful. She has tried a variety of pain pills without any help. She tried Mycostatin at the onset without any benefit. She has been treated with triamcinolone dental paste without any benefit. She does not have any dentures.

There is a medical history of hyperlipidemia on colesevelam (Welchol) and mild depression on buproprion (Wellbutrin). Oropharyngeal and neurologic examinations were normal. Serum zinc, ferritin, and vitamin B_{12} levels were normal. Complete blood count and glycosylated hemoglobin was normal. Sjögren antibodies were negative [32].

Questions

What is the diagnosis? Which treatments are available?

Discussion

Burning mouth syndrome is characterized by a burning, tingling, hot, scalded, or numb sensation in the oral cavity in patients who have a clinically normal oral mucosal examination [33]. Synonyms include glossodynia, glossopyrosis, glossalgia, stomatodynia, stomatopyrosis, sore tongue and mouth, burning tongue, oral or lingual paresthesia, and oral dysesthesia. This pain occurs most commonly on the anterior two thirds and tip of the tongue but also may occur on the upper alveolar region, palate, lips, and lower alveolar region. Less commonly, the buccal muscosa, floor of the mouth, and the throat are affected. The pain may be constant or absent in the morning and progress during the day or be intermittent with symptom-free intervals. The prevalence in the general population is 3.7% with a 7:1 female-to-male ratio, usually in a middle-aged and elderly population, with a mean age of 60 years. Burning mouth syndrome, thus, is not an uncommon disorder but is one that may be uncommonly seen and recognized by neurologists.

The diagnosis is one of exclusion. Although approximately one third may have a psychiatric disorder, often depression, anxiety, or other causes should be considered. The following are causes: xerostomia or dry mouth, which can be the result of medications, such as tricyclic antidepressants, or systemic disease, such as Sjögren's; nutritional deficiency, such as iron, vitamin B_{12}, zinc, or B-complex vitamins; a trigeminal small fiber neuropathy [34]; allergic contact dermatitis resulting from food and oral preparation, which may be detected by patch testing; denture-related etiology; parafunctional behavior, such as clenching or grind the teeth, thrusting the tongue, or running the tongue along the teeth. Candidiasis may be a cause in up to 30% of cases and can be present with a normal examination; diabetes mellitus may be present in 5% of cases; and angiotensin-converting enzyme inhibitors (eg, enalapril, captropril, and lisinopril) can be a cause.

If an underlying cause cannot be found and treated, treatments that might be tried include empiric anticandidal agents, B-complex vitamins, tricyclic antidepressants, gabapentin, oral clonazepam, and topical clonazepam (sucking a 1-mg tablet for 3 minutes and then spitting it out 3 times a day) [35,36]. Women who are postmenopausal might benefit from estrogen-progesterone replacement therapy [37].

Case 8. Headache triggered by straining, stooping, or getting up from a sitting position

This is a 66-year-old white man who has had occasional mild headaches in the past. He presented with a 4-month history of headaches occurring 1 to 4 times per day, brought on by having a bowel movement, stooping, or getting up from a sitting position. He did not know if the headaches were triggered by coughing, because he had not coughed at all. The headaches were a bifrontal and bitemporal sharp, aching pain with a 7/10 intensity and occasionally a 9/10 intensity, with an average duration of 1 minute and a range of 30 seconds to 1 hour. Approximately 20 of the headaches had lasted more than 1 minute, with most in a range of 1 to 2 minutes. He had tried ibuprofen and acetaminophen with questionable help. For the prior 5 days, he had increased his dose of aspirin from 81 mg per day to 325 mg per day. The headache then was different with a constant bifrontotemporal pressure with an intensity of 1/10 but he had not had the brief headaches with activity exacerbation. He had a CT scan of the sinuses on June 14, 2004, with essentially negative findings.

There was a medical history of insulin-dependent diabetes with sensory neuropathy and hypertension. Neurologic examination was normal except for diminished pinprick distally of both lower extremities and absent deep tendon reflexes diffusely.

MRI scan of the brain was normal except for smooth diffuse dural enhancement around both cerebral convexities and, to a milder degree, in the posterior fossa. A lumbar puncture produced an opening pressure of 11 cm of water. Cerebrospinal fluid (CSF) analysis revealed 0 white blood cells, 1 red blood cell/µL, a glucose of 101 mg/dL (with a serum glucose of 156 mg/dL), and a protein of 109 mg/dL. The VDRL was nonreactive. An erythrocyte sedimentation rate was [36]. ANA, rheumatoid arthritis (RA) factor, Sjögren's antibodies, Lyme antibodies, and angiotensin-converting enzyme level were negative or normal. MRI scan of the cervical, thoracic, and lumbar spine revealed degenerative changes but no evidence of extra-arachnoid fluid collections, extradural extravasation of fluid, or meningeal diverticula.

Questions

What is the diagnosis? What are the MRI findings in this disorder?

Discussion

The history could be compatible with primary cough headache as defined by the International Headache Society's second edition criteria: sudden onset, lasting from 1 second to 30 minutes, and brought on by and occurring only in association with coughing, straining, or Valsalva's maneuver [38]. Primary cough headache, however, is a diagnosis of exclusion, where the symptoms cannot be attributed to another disorder. Primary cough headache usually is bilateral and affects predominantly patients older than 40. In some cases, the onset may be after a respiratory infection with cough. The term, cough headache, also is used by many to include headaches brought on by sneezing, weightlifting, bending, stooping, or straining with a bowel movement. Weightlifting also can cause an acute bilateral nuchal-occipital or nuchal-occipital-parietal headache that can persist as a residual ache for days or weeks, which may be the result of stretching of cervical ligaments and tendons. Other secondary causes should be excluded as appropriate, such as subarachnoid hemorrhage. Although primary cough headache is associated with an increase in intracranial pressure, the exact cause of the pain is not certain. Posterior cranial fossa overcrowding may be a contributing factor [8].

Primary cough headache may be diagnosed only after structural lesions are excluded, such as posterior fossa tumor, Chiari I malformation, platybasia, basilar impression, spontaneous intracranial hypotension (SIH), pneumocephalus, middle cranial fossa or posterior fossa meningioma, medulloblastoma, pinealoma, chromophobe adenoma, midbrain cyst, and subdural hematoma (excluded by neuroimaging) [39]. Internal carotid artery stenosis and unruptured intracranial saccular aneurysms are questionable associations with unilateral cough headache. MRI of the brain without and with contrast is the preferred imaging study to exclude secondary causes.

Benign cough headaches (and less often secondary cases) may respond to indomethacin (25–50 mg 3 times a day) [9], lumbar puncture [10], methysergide [11], acetazolamide (500–2000 mg per day in divided doses) [12], and perhaps topiramate (because of its weak carbonic anhydrase inhibition). Some patients may have an abrupt recovery after extraction of abscessed teeth.

SIH syndrome often presents with a headache when upright, which is relieved by lying down, or an orthostatic headache. As SIH persists, however, chronic daily headaches may be present without orthostatic features. SIH also may present with other types of headaches, including exertional without any orthostatic features, acute thunderclap onset, parodoxic orthostatic headaches (present in recumbency and relieved when upright), intermittent headaches resulting from intermittent leaks, and the acephalgic form (no headaches). Neck or interscapular pain may precede the onset of headaches in some cases by days or weeks.

Box 1 summarizes MRI abnormalities of the brain and spine that are variably present. SIH can be present with a normal MRI with contrast of the brain and spine. MRI scan of the brain may reveal diffuse pachymeningeal (dural) enhancement with gadolinium without leptomeningeal (arachnoid

---

Box 1. MRI abnormalities in cerebrospinal fluid leaks

Head MRI
Diffuse pachymeningeal (dural) enhancement
Descent ("sagging" or "sinking") of the brain
- Descent of cerebellar tonsils (may mimic type I Chiari)
- Obliteration of some of the subarachnoid cisterns (ie, prepontine or perichiasmatic cisterns)
- Crowding of the posterior fossa
Enlargement of the pituitary
Flattening or "tenting" of the optic chiasm
Subdural fluid collections (typically hygromas, infrequently hematomas)
Engorged cerebral venous sinuses
Decrease in size of the ventricles (ventricular collapse)
Increase in anteroposterior diameter of the brainstem

Spine MRI
Extra-arachnoid fluid collections (often extending across several levels)
Extradural extravasation of fluid (extending to paraspinal soft tissues)
Meningeal diverticula
Identification of level of the leak (not uncommonly)
Identification of the actual site of the leak (very uncommonly)
Spinal pachymeningeal enhancement
Engorgement of spinal epidural venous plexus

From Mokri B. Low cerebrospinal fluid pressure syndromes. Neurol Clin North Am 2004;22:55–74; with permission.

and pial) involvement and, in some cases, subdural fluid collections, which return to normal with resolution of the headache. One is reversible descent of the cerebellar tonsils below the foramen magnum (acquired Chiari I malformation), which can be the result of SIH and also the result of lumbar puncture and overdraining CSF shunts. The diffuse meningeal enhancement on MRI may be explained by dural vasodilation and a greater concentration of gadolinium in the dural microvasculature and in the interstitial fluid of the dura. (Before the characteristic picture of the postural headache and diffuse pachymeningeal enhancement on MRI was recognized, some patients underwent extensive testing, including meningeal biopsy, to exclude other conditions, such as meningeal carcinomatosis and neurosarcoidosis.) The pleocytosis and elevated protein in the CSF and the subdural fluid collections probably are the result of decreased CSF volume and hydrostatic pressure changes resulting in meningeal vasodilation and vascular leak.

A lumbar puncture usually demonstrates an opening pressure from 0 to 70 cm H_2O (and can even be negative), although the pressure can be in the normal range, especially if the procedure is performed after a period of bed rest. The CSF analysis may be normal or can demonstrate a moderate, primarily lymphocytic pleocytosis (50 cells/mm^3 are common and values may be as high as 220 cells/mm^3), the presence of red blood cells, and elevated protein levels that rarely are as high as 1000 mg/dL. CSF glucose concentration never is low.

CT myelography is more sensitive than other studies for determining the actual site of a CSF leak, because most leaks occur in the spine, especially at the thoracic level. Because the leaks can be high or low flow, early and delayed CT may be helpful. The study may demonstrate extra-arachnoid fluid, meningeal diverticula, and extradural leak of contrast into the paraspinal soft tissues.

Radioisotope cisternography using indium 111 may demonstrate an absence or paucity of activity over the cerebral convexities at 24 or 48 hours. Less commonly, parathecal activity at the approximate level of the leak may be apparent.

Case 9. Headache with walking

Grace and colleagues report the following case:

A 59-year-old man presented to the hospital neurosurgical department with a history of severe headache experienced in all of the vertex and upper occipital area on exercise. Before this presentation there was no history of significant or persistent headache. The pain appeared immediately on walking at a normal pace and immediately was relieved on rest. It was described as bursting in quality and severe in degree. There was no history of chest pain.

Resting electrocardiograph (ECG) revealed T-wave inversion in the anterolateral leads. Treadmill exercise immediately induced the same headache in the same location. The headache was severe and associated with simultaneous further S-T depression on the ECG. The headache and the fresh S-T segment abnormality resolved immediately with rest. Coronary angiography revealed two areas of subtotal occlusion at the midpoint of the right coronary. There also was 70% stenosis of the left anterior descending coronary artery (LAD) proximal to the diagonal branch [40].

He underwent aortocoronary bypass surgery and was headache-free for 7 years. The same exertional headache recurred with resolution following angioplasty of a high-grade stenosis of the LAD. One year later, an exertional headache recurred that did not resolve despite repeat bypass surgery and was believed the result of refractory cardiac ischemia.

Questions

Which types of headaches are associated with exertion? What is the diagnosis? What is the mechanism for the referred head pain?

Discussion

Primary (benign) exertional headache, which has a lifetime prevalence of 1% [41], is brought on by and occurs only during or after physical exercise and lasts from 5 minutes to 48 hours [39]. It typically is a throbbing bilateral headache and not attributed to another cause. Reported activities include running, rowing, tennis, and swimming. One particular activity may precipitate the headaches in some individuals but not others. This headache type is prevented by avoiding excessive exertion, particularly in hot weather or at high altitude. Exercise can be a trigger for a typical migraine for some migraineurs. Secondary causes to be excluded include subarachnoid hemorrhage (SAH), pheochromocytomas, cardiac ischemia, middle cerebral artery dissection, paranasal sinusitis, intracranial neoplasms, colloid cysts of the third ventricle, and hypoplasia of the aortic arch after successful coarctation repair. An MRI of the brain with magnetic resonance angiography assists in ruling out structural or vascular lesions.

In some cases, exertional headaches may be prevented by a warm-up period. Some patients choose to avoid the particular activity. Indomethacin (25–150 mg per day) may work as a preventive, taken minutes to 1 hour before exertion. Prophylactic drugs used for migraine, such as β-blockers, may be effective for some patients.

Cardiac ischemia rarely may cause a unilateral or bilateral headache in any part of the head brought on by exercise and relieved by rest, cardiac cephalalgia, or anginal headache [42,43]. Headaches rarely may occur alone or be accompanied by chest pain. In cases of unstable angina, headaches may occur at rest [44].

Angina generally is believed the result of afferent impulses that traverse cervicothoracic sympathetic ganglia, enter the spinal cord via the first and the fifth thoracic dorsal roots, and produce the characteristic pain in the chest or inner aspects of the arms. Cardiac vagal afferents, which mediate anginal pain in a minority of patients, join the tractus solitarius. Although the cause is not known, a potential pathway for referral of cardiac pain to the head would be convergence with craniovascular afferents [45]. Two other possible mechanisms of headache are suggested [42]. A reduction of cardiac output and an increase in right atrial pressure occur in myocardial ischemia. The associated reduction in venous return may increase intracranial pressure, which could produce headache. Second, release of chemical mediators resulting from myocardial ischemia (serotonin, bradykinin, histamine, and substance P) may stimulate nociceptive intracranial receptors and produce headache.

References

[1] Evans RW, Pearce JMS. Exploding head syndrome. Headache 2001;41:602–3.
[2] Pearce JM. Exploding head syndrome. Lancet 1988;2:270–1.
[3] Peres MFP. Sleep disorders associated with headaches. In: Gilman S, editor. MedLink neurology. San Diego: MedLink Corp; 2006. Available at www.medlink.com. Accessed February 10, 2006.
[4] Evans RW, Dodick DW, Schwedt TJ. Headache causing awakening from sleep. Headache, in press.
[5] Raskin NH. Raskin NH. The hypnic headache syndrome. Headache 1988;28:534–6.
[6] Grosberg BM, Lipton RB, Solomon S, et al. Hypnic headache in childhood? A case report. Cephalalgia 2004;25:68–70.
[7] Evers S, Goadsby PJ. Hypnic headache: clinical features, pathophysiology, and treatment. Neurology 2003;60:905–9.
[8] Dodick DW. Polysomnography in Hypnic Headache Syndrome. Headache 2000;40:748–52.
[9] Peatfield RC, Mendoza ND. Posterior fossa meningioma presenting as hypnic headache. Headache 2003;43:1007–8.
[10] Evans RW, Lance JW. Transient headache with numbness of half of the tongue. Headache 2000;40:692–3.
[11] Lance JW, Anthony M. Neck-tongue syndrome on sudden turning of the head. J Neurol Neurosurg Psychiatry 1980;43:97–101.
[12] Lewis DW, Frank LM, Toor S. Familial neck-tongue syndrome. Headache 2003;43:132–4.
[13] Evans RW, Rolak LA. The Alice in Wonderland Syndrome. Headache 2004;44:624–5.
[14] Evans RW. Reversible palinposia and the Alice in Wonderland associated with topiramate use in migraineurs. Headache 2006; in press.
[15] Lippman CW. Certain hallucinations peculiar to migraine. J Nerve Mental Dis 1952;116:346.
[16] Todd J. The syndrome of Alice in Wonderland. Can Med Assoc J 1955;73:701.
[17] Rolak LA. Literary neurologic syndromes. Alice in Wonderland. Arch Neurol 1991;48:649–51.
[18] Restak RM. Alice in Migraineland. Headache 2006; in press.
[19] Liu GT, Volpe NJ, Galetta SL. Visual hallucinations and illusions. Neuro-ophthalmology. Diagnosis and management. Philadelphia: WB Saunders; 2001. p. 401–24.
[20] Evens RW, Pareja JA. Nummular headache. Headache 2005;45:164–5.
[21] Pareja JA, Pareja J, Yangüela J. Nummular headache, trochleitis, supraorbital neuralgia, and other epicranial headaches and neuralgias: the epicranias. J Headache Pain 2003;4:125–31.

[22] Pareja JA, Caminero AB, Serra J, et al. Numular headache: a coin-shaped cephalgia. Neurology 2002;58:1678–9.

[23] Pareja JA, Pareja J, Barriga FJ, et al. Nummular headache: a prospective series of 14 new cases. Headache 2004;44:611–4.

[24] Cohen GL. Nummular headache: what denomination? Headache 2005;10:1417–8.

[25] Evans RW, Lance JW. The red ear syndrome: an auriculo-autonomic cephalgia. Headache 2004;44:835–6.

[26] Lance JW. The mystery of one red ear. Clin Exp Neurol 1995;31:13–8.

[27] Al-Din AS, Mir R, Davey R, et al. Trigeminal cephalgias and facial pain syndromes associated with autonomic dysfunction. Cephalalgia 2005;25:605–11.

[28] Raieli V, Monastero R, Santangelo G, et al. Red ear syndrome and migraine: report of eight cases. Headache 2002;42:147–51.

[29] Lance JW. The red ear syndrome. Neurology 1996;47:617–20.

[30] Kumar N, Swanson JW. The 'red ear syndrome' revisited: two cases and a review of literature. Cephalalgia 2004;24:305–8.

[31] Arjona A, Serrano-Castro PJ, Fernandez-Romero E, et al. The red ear syndrome: five new cases. Cephalalgia 2005;25:479–80.

[32] Evans RW, Drage LA. Burning mouth syndrome. Headache 2005;45:1079–81.

[33] Drage LA, Rogers RS. Burning mouth syndrome. Dermatol Clin 2003;21:135–45.

[34] Lauria G, Majorana A, Borgna M, et al. Trigeminal small-fiber sensory neuropathy causes burning mouth syndrome. Pain 2005;115:332–7.

[35] Gremeau-Richard C, Woda A, Navez ML, et al. Topical clonazepam in stomatodynia: a randomised placebo-controlled study. Pain 2004;108:51–7.

[36] Zakrzewska JM, Forssell H, Glenny AM. Interventions for the treatment of burning mouth syndrome. Cochrane Database Syst Rev 2005;1:CD002779.

[37] Santoro V, Caputo G, Peluso F. Clinical and therapeutic experience in twenty eight patients with burning mouth syndrome. Minerva Stomatol 2005;54:489–96.

[38] Headache Classification Subcommittee of the International Headache Society. The International Classification of Headache Disorders. 2nd ed. Cephalalgia 2004;24(Suppl 1):1–160.

[39] Cutrer FM, Boes CJ. Cough, exertional, and sex headaches. Neurol Clin North Am 2004;22: 133–49.

[40] Grace A, Horgan J, Breathnach K, et al. Anginal headache and its basis. Cephalalgia 1997; 17:195–6.

[41] Rasmussen BK, Olesen J. Symptomatic and nonsymptomatic headaches in a general population. Neurology 1992;42:1225–31.

[42] Lipton RB, Lowenkopf T, Bajwa ZH, et al. Cardiac cephalalgia: a treatable form of exertional headache. Neurology 1997;49:813–6.

[43] Sathirapanya P. Anginal cephalgia: a serious form of exertional headache. Cephalalgia 2004; 24:231–4.

[44] Lanza GA, Sciahbasi A, Sestito A, et al. Angina pectoris: a headache. Lancet 2000; 16;356:998.

[45] Lance JW, Lambros J. Unilateral exertional headache as a symptom of cardiac ischemia. Headache 1998;38:315–6.

ELSEVIER
SAUNDERS

Neurol Clin 24 (2006) 363–369

NEUROLOGIC
CLINICS

Psychosis in Parkinson's Disease: Case Studies

Brian C. Salter, MD[a], Karen E. Anderson, MD[a,b,*], William J. Weiner, MD[a,c]

[a]Department of Neurology, University of Maryland School of Medicine, Baltimore, MD, USA
[b]Department of Psychiatry, University of Maryland School of Medicine, Baltimore, MD, USA
[c]Parkinson's and Movement Disorders Center, University of Maryland, Baltimore, MD, USA

Hallucinations and psychotic symptoms are common in patients who have Parkinson's disease (PD), affecting a third of patients who have PD at some point during the illness. Psychotic symptoms are related to several factors, including the underlying disease process, concurrent difficulties with visual impairment and sleep disturbance, and adverse effects of dopaminergic agents used to treat the movement disorder. Psychosis in patients who have PD leads to higher hospitalization rates, significantly increased disability, nursing home placement, and increased risk of mortality. Treatment involves education, development of patient coping strategies, modification of the PD drug regimen, or the addition of an antipsychotic agent, such as quetiapine, or, in more refractory cases, clozapine.

Cases

Case 1

A 70-year-old woman diagnosed with levodopa-responsive PD 10 years previously was brought in by her family for a follow-up visit with her neurologist. She was not experiencing motor fluctuations or dyskinesias and she was satisfied with current control of her motor symptoms. During

* Corresponding author. Room N4W46, Movement Disorders Division, Department of Neurology, University of Maryland, School of Medicine, 22 South Greene Street, Baltimore, MD 21201.
  E-mail address: kanderson@psych.umaryland.edu (K.E. Anderson).

0733-8619/06/$ - see front matter © 2006 Elsevier Inc. All rights reserved.
doi:10.1016/j.ncl.2006.01.003
neurologic.theclinics.com

the visit, one of her children remarked that the mother's "leprechauns had been coming out more than usual in the last weeks." The family explained that the patient had been seeing small people dressed in fancy costumes sitting in her living room for the last few months. She noticed them when she came downstairs in the morning for breakfast. The patient was embarrassed at having this revealed to her doctor but denied any distress resulting from these hallucinations. She and her children insisted she always was aware they were not real; she found them to be amusing.

Questions
What is the diagnosis? What is the etiology?

Comment
This patient has mild visual hallucinations related to her antiparkinsonian drug regimen. Psychotic symptoms are common in PD, affecting approximately one third of patients. These symptoms include hallucinations, psychosis, and delusions. Approximately half of patients who have hallucinations have pure visual hallucinations [1]; auditory, mixed, tactile, and olfactory hallucinations are less common [2,3].

Diederich and colleagues propose a new theoretic model for hallucinations in PD as a dysregulation of processing external stimuli and creating an internal image [4]. This dysregulation is believed the result of several factors, including decreased visual acuity, aberrant activation of the frontal cortex, intrusion of rapid eye movement (REM) sleep, and overstimulation of the mesolimbic dopamine system. Positron emission tomography studies suggest that patients who have visual hallucinations have an abnormal increase in metabolism in the frontal lobe and other anterior regions [5,6].

Psychosis typically does not occur early in PD. If it does, the underlying diagnosis should be questioned. Most patients diagnosed with PD who have early-onset hallucinations (ie, within the first year) actually have a different underlying disorder, such as Lewy body disease or a pre-existing psychiatric condition [7].

Sleep disorders can contribute to psychosis. Patients may have disrupted sleep, impaired REM sleep, or REM sleep behavior disorder making them more susceptible to hallucinations [1,8–11]. Visual system abnormalities likely contribute to visual hallucinations [12]. Patients who have PD may have ocular changes, such as decreased blink rate and retinal abnormalities [13]. Cognitive impairment, dementia, and psychiatric comorbidities, such as depression and anxiety, also may contribute to psychosis. Psychotic symptoms are reported after surgical treatments for PD [14–16].

Adverse drug effects are a major contributing factor to psychosis. The majority of hallucinations are related to agents used to treat PD. Saint-Cyr and coworkers reviewed the psychiatric side effects of pharmacologic therapy for PD and found that levodopa is associated with an approximately 20% incidence of hallucinations [14]. Combination therapy with levodopa and pergolide increase the incidence to approximately 30% [17].

Amantadine may cause hallucinations and confusion, particularly in patients over age 65 [18]. Symptoms may vary with the timing of drug administration; nighttime administration of dopaminergic drugs often is associated with the presence of psychotic symptoms [19].

Treatment of psychosis in PD is individualized and may include several components. If symptoms are not disturbing and are tolerable, observation is recommended (especially if insight is preserved, as in Case 1). Patient coping strategies may be useful; Diederich and colleagues found that approximately 80% of patients who have PD with visual hallucinations use coping strategies [20]. These strategies are divided into cognitive, inter-active, and visual techniques. Cognitive techniques include reassurance that the hallucinations are not real and self-initiated reactions, such as turning on the lights. Interactive techniques include attempting to touch the hallucina-tions to ensure they are not real. Visual techniques include looking away, focusing on a different object, and focusing better on the hallucination [20].

If these strategies are insufficient, the next level of management is to mod-ify the PD medication regimen. Withdrawal of the most recently added agent often is sufficient, especially if a medication change preceded the onset of psychosis. In some cases, a dose reduction may be all that is needed. If hallucinations persist, all medications a patient is taking, in particular the antiparkinsonian agents, may need to be removed. Each medication must be assessed regarding its potential risk/benefit ratio with respect to the hallucinations/motor benefit ratio. Subsequently, medications need to be withdrawn until unacceptable motor consequences develop. Some nonphar-macologic approaches include improved lighting and corrective lenses. Comorbidities, such as depression, anxiety, and dementia, should be treated. If patients have persistent troubling psychosis even after these interventions, the next step is the addition of an antipsychotic agent. Atypical antipsychotics are preferred because they are less likely to worsen motor function. Use of these agents is discussed in detail after Case 2.

Case 2

A 49-year-old man who had a 5-year history of PD was brought to the clinic by his family because of persistent thoughts that his neighbors had placed him under surveillance. His PD was being treated with carbidopa/levodopa (25/250-mg tablets, one every 4 hours) and pramipexole (1.5 mg every 8 hours). One year ago he had surgical placement of a deep brain stimulator (DBS) for treatment of motor symptoms. Two weeks after stimulation be-gan, he developed paranoia that his neighbors were monitoring his every move. After a verbal altercation with a neighbor, whom he accused of spying on him, he was taken to an emergency department by police. On questioning at the emergency department, the patient's family reported he had been very suspicious of the neighbors before DBS surgery, occasionally asking if "they were watching our house or if our phone was tapped." He had not acted on the suspicions before the surgery, however, so the family had not reported them to anyone. Quetiapine (25 mg) was started and he was referred to his neurologist. At the time of the current assessment, he was taking carbidopa/levodopa (25/250-mg tablets every 4 hours), pramipexole (1.5 mg every 8 hours), and quetiapine (25 mg) every evening.

Questions

What is the diagnosis? What is the etiology?

Comment

Visual hallucinations can be formed or nonformed and threatening or nonthreatening. Patients who have hallucinations have a continuum of insight, ranging from full insight, as in Case 1, to partial insight to a complete lack of insight [12]. Patients develop delusions or even frank psychosis when insight is lost. The patient in Case 2 had delusions and paranoia. Some patients may act on their hallucinations or delusions, as this patient did when he confronted his neighbor.

The cause of the psychosis in Case 2 likely is multifactorial. In this patient, the psychotic symptoms did not receive clinical attention until after the DBS surgery, although he had paranoia before this. His family reported that he had periods of paranoia before DBS when dopaminergic agents were administered at higher doses. He also had a history of psychiatric comorbidity with depression and anxiety, both of which previously were treated pharmacologically.

Question

What is the management approach?

Comment

When he was brought to the emergency department by the police, the patient was admitted to a psychiatric unit for evaluation and treatment of psychosis. An emergency department or inpatient evaluation may be needed for new onset of hallucinations, particularly if the patient is violent or uncontrollable. Most patients who have PD and psychosis, however, can be evaluated and treated as outpatients. In more severe cases, such as the patient in case 2, a locked psychiatric inpatient unit is the safest place to begin treatment. A locked unit with a high level of individual patient monitoring is preferable for patients who have severe psychopathology to prevent them from escaping, harming themselves, or acting aggressively toward others if they believe they are in danger. In some instances, new-onset hallucinations can be precipitated by sepsis, in particular pneumonia or a urinary tract infection.

Having patients and caregivers meet together often is helpful. Physicians can facilitate discussion about the character and implications of hallucinations and delusions. Often, patients have developed their own coping strategies, such as touching a figure to see if it is real, because the visual hallucinations seen by patients who have PD often disappear when patients attempt to interact with them. It is useful to identify these and discuss them with patients and caregivers. Caregivers often are reassured by these discussions.

This patient was not having hallucinations at the time of the interview in clinic. He also denied having delusions at that time, saying he did not believe his house was under surveillance. Thus, he used cognitive coping strategies most of the time, reminding himself that the delusions were not real. He qualified this, however, by saying that when he was having episodes of paranoia they seemed extremely real, and, at those times, he believed that he was unable to tell if his house was under surveillance or not.

When patient coping strategies are insufficient, the next step is to adjust the antiparkinsonian drug regimen. When this patient later developed an acute episode of paranoia, the dopamine agonist was discontinued. In some cases, when psychosis is associated with DBS, the DBS parameters may need to be adjusted. Another important aspect of management is to address comorbidities. This patient also had depression, anxiety, and difficulty sleeping; a selective serotonin reuptake inhibitor was started to help reduce anxiety about the delusions, and a sleeping medication was added later (escitalopram and trazadone, respectively).

If patients have persistent debilitating psychotic symptoms, an antipsychotic medication may be required. Atypical antipsychotics are the preferred agents for treatment of patients who have PD. Quetiapine is efficacious in treating PD psychosis, usually without worsening motor symptoms [21–26] and is the atypical antipsychotic medication most widely used for this purpose by movement disorder specialists. This patient started quetiapine. Quetiapine should be started at a low dose (such as 12.5 mg each evening) and increased gradually to minimize side effects. In patients who have PD, doses higher than 75 mg per day seldom are required. The patient developed fatigue, a common side effect of quetiapine. He did not have any worsening motor symptoms.

If psychotic symptoms persist or side effects limit quetiapine administration, switch to clozapine. Most patients who do not respond to quetiapine have a favorable response with clozapine. Several open-label studies demonstrated that clozapine is effective in treating psychosis in patients who have PD [27–29]. The Parkinson Study Group showed significant benefit with clozapine in a randomized, double-blind, placebo-controlled trial [30]. Clozapine therapy requires close monitoring of complete blood count because of a 1% to 2% incidence of agranulocytosis. Patients also must be registered in the National Clozapine Database. This usually limits its use to tertiary centers. Risperdone and olanzapine are not used for psychosis in patients who have PD, because, although they may improve psychosis, motor function often is worsened significantly [24,31–34].

Clinicians should be aware of recent Food and Drug Administration warnings that use of atypical antipsychotics is associated with an increased risk of death in a review of data from 5106 elderly demented patients in randomized controlled clinical trials [35]. A mortality rate of 4.5% was seen in those elders receiving atypicals compared with 2.6% in those given placebo. Deaths predominantly were the result of cardiovascular and infectious illnesses. A black-box warning has been added to labeling of all atypical neuroleptics, calling attention to these findings. Many of the patients who are most in need of treatment for behavioral side effects of PD medications are elderly and may have memory loss; thus, they may be at higher risk of mortality associated with atypical neuroleptic use. As discussed previously, the presence of psychotic symptoms in PD is associated with significant risk of increased morbidity and mortality. Clinicians should weigh carefully the small possibility of increased mortality associated with atypical antipsychotic use versus the many complications inherent in leaving psychotic symptoms untreated in these patients.

Summary

Psychosis is common in patients who have PD and leads to significant disability. Patients often can be managed with nonpharmacologic interventions or with decreasing doses of antiparkinsonism medications. If these interventions are insufficient, then atypical antipsychotics should be considered. Clozapine is used in more refractory cases and requires stringent monitoring for agranulocytosis.

References

[1] Goetz CG, Wuu J, Curgian LM, et al. Hallucinations and sleep disorders in PD. Neurology 2005;64:81–6.
[2] Inzelberg R, Kipervasser S, Korczyn AD. Auditory hallucinations in Parkinson's disease. J Neurol Neurosurg Psychiatry 1998;64:533–5.
[3] Fenelon G, Mahieux F, Huon R, et al. Hallucinations in Parkinson's disease: prevalence, phenomenology and risk factors. Brain 2000;124:733–45.
[4] Diederich NJ, Goetz CG, Stebbins GT. Repeated visual hallucinations in Parkinson's disease as disturbed external/internal perceptions: focused review and a new integrative model. Mov Disord 2005;20:130–40.
[5] Nagano-Saito A, Washimi Y, Arahata Y, et al. Visual hallucination in Parkinson's disease with FDG PET. Mov Disord 2004;19:801–6.
[6] Stebbins GT, Goetz CG, Carrillo MC, et al. Altered cortical visual processing in PD with hallucinations: an fMRI study. Neurology 2004;63:1409–16.
[7] Goetz CG, Vogel C, Tanner CM, et al. Early dopaminergic drug-induced hallucinations in Parkinsonian patients. Neurology 1998;51:811–4.
[8] Comella CL, Tanner CM, Ristanovic RK. Polysomnographic sleep measures in Parkinson's disease patients with treatment-induced hallucinations. Ann Neurol 1993;34:710–4.
[9] Rye DB, Bliwise DL, Dihenia B, et al. Daytime sleepiness in Parkinson's disease. J Sleep Res 2000;9:63–9.
[10] Arnulf I, Bonnet AM, Damier P, et al. Hallucinations, REM sleep, and Parkinson's disease: a medical hypothesis. Neurology 2000;55:281–8.

[11] Nomura T, Inoue Y, Mitani H, et al. Visual hallucinations as REM sleep behavior disorders in patients with Parkinson's disease. Mov Disord 2003;18:812–7.

[12] Holroyd S, Currie L, Wooten GF. Prospective study of hallucinations and delusions in Parkinson's disease. J Neurol Neurosurg Psychiatry 2001;70:734–8.

[13] Biousse V, Skibell BC, Watts RL, et al. Ophthalmologic features of Parkinson's disease. Neurology 2004;62:177–80.

[14] Saint-Cyr JA, Taylor AE, Lang AE. Neuropsychological and psychiatric side effects in the treatment of Parkinson's disease. Neurology 1993;43(Suppl 6):S47–52.

[15] Kulisevsky J, Berthier ML, Gironell A, et al. Mania following deep brain stimulation for Parkinson's disease. Neurology 2002;59:1421–4.

[16] Diederich NJ, Alesch F, Goetz CG. Visual hallucinations induced by deep brain stimulation in Parkinson's disease. Clin Neuropharmacol 2000;23:287–9.

[17] Jankovic J. Long-term study of pergolide in Parkinson's disease. Neurology 1985;35:296–9.

[18] Timberlake WH, Vance MA. Four-year treatment of patients with Parkinsonism using amantadine alone or with levodopa. Ann Neurol 1978;3:119–28.

[19] Juncos JL. Management of psychotic aspects of Parkinson's disease. J Clin Psychiatry 1999; 60(Suppl 8):42–53.

[20] Diederich NJ, Pieri V, Goetz CG. Coping strategies for visual hallucinations in Parkinson's disease. Mov Disord 2003;18:831–2.

[21] Fernandez HH, Friedman JH, Jacques C, et al. Quetiapine for the treatment of drug-induced psychosis in Parkinson's disease. Mov Disord 1999;14:484–7.

[22] Juncos JL, Arvanitis L, Sweitzer D, et al. Quetiapine improves psychotic symptoms associated with Parkinson's disease. Neurology 1999;52:A262.

[23] Dewey RB, O'Suilleabhain PE. Treatment of drug-induced psychosis with quetiapine and clozapine in Parkinson's disease. Neurology 2000;55:1753–4.

[24] Weiner WJ, Minagar A, Shulman LM. Quetiapine for L-dopa-induced psychosis in PD. Neurology 2000;54:1538.

[25] Brandstadter D, Oertel WH. Treatment of drug-induced psychosis with quetiapine and clozapine in Parkinson's disease. Neurology 2002;58:160–1.

[26] Fernandez HH, Trieschmann ME, Burke MA, et al. Long-term outcome of quetiapine use for psychosis among Parkinsonian patients. Mov Disord 2003;18:510–4.

[27] Friedman JH, Lannon MC. Clozapine in the treatment of psychosis in Parkinson's disease. Neurology 1989;39:1219–21.

[28] Factor SA, Brown D, Molho ES, et al. Clozapine: a 2-year open trial in Parkinson's disease patients with psychosis. Neurology 1994;44:544–6.

[29] Wagner ML, Defilippi JL, Menza MA, et al. Clozapine for the treatment of psychosis in Parkinson's disease: chart review of 49 patients. J Neuropsychiatry Clin Neurosci 1996;8: 276–80.

[30] Parkinson Study Group. Low-dose clozapine for the treatment of drug-induced psychosis in Parkinson's disease. N Engl J Med 1999;340:757–63.

[31] Graham JM, Sussman JD, Ford KS, et al. Olanzapine in the treatment of hallucinosis in idiopathic Parkinson's disease: a cautionary note. J Neurol Neurosurg Psychiatry 1998;65: 774–7.

[32] Ellis T, Cudkowicz ME, Sexton PM, et al. Clozapine and risperidone treatment of psychosis in Parkinson's disease. J Neuropsychiatry Clin Neurosci 2000;12:364–9.

[33] Goetz CG, Blasucci LM, Leurgans S, et al. Olanzapine and clozapine: comparative effects on motor function in hallucinating PD patients. Neurology 2000;55:789–94.

[34] Marsh L, Lyketsos C, Reich SG. Olanzapine for the treatment of psychosis in patients with Parkinson's disease and dementia. Psychosomatics 2001;42:477–81.

[35] Kuehn BM. FDA warns antipsychotic drugs may be risky for elderly. JAMA 2005;293: 22462.

Neuromuscular Disorders in Medical and Surgical ICUs: Case Studies in Critical Care Neurology

Boby Varkey Maramattom, MD, DM,
Eelco F.M. Wijdicks, MD*

*Division of Critical Care Neurology, Department of Neurology,
Mayo Clinic College of Medicine, Rochester, MN, USA*

Patients either can be admitted to critical care unit with generalized weakness or develop weakness de novo in ICUs. This comorbidity prolongs hospital stay, increases morbidity and mortality, and inflates hospital costs by thousands of dollars [1].

With advances in supportive care, critical care, and antibiotic therapy, the mortality rate in ICUs has improved steadily during the past few decades. As a result, the spectrum of neuromuscular disease in today's ICUs also has evolved during the past few decades. Nowadays, de novo weakness in ICUs (such as critical illness myopathy [CIM] or polyneuropathy [CIP]) is 2 to 3 times more common than primary neuromuscular disorders, such as Guillain-Barré syndrome (GBS), myopathies, or motor neuron disease [2].

Patients in ICUs can develop a variety of mononeuropathies or plexopathies related to ischemia, pressure palsies, prolonged recumbency, compartment syndromes, or hematoma. They also can develop weakness resulting from intracranial processes. It is estimated that almost 12% of patients in medical ICUs experience a neurologic complication. These patients have a higher mortality rate and experience a longer stay in an ICU [3]. The most common neurologic complications are metabolic encephalopathy, seizures, hypoxic-ischemic encephalopathy, and stroke. Some of these conditions can present with generalized weakness. Nonetheless, generalized weakness in ICUs is associated more commonly with neuromuscular or

---

* Corresponding author. Mayo Clinic College of Medicine, Division of Critical Care Neurology, Department of Neurology, W8B, 200 First Street SW, Rochester, MN 55905.

E-mail address: wijde@mayo.edu (E.F.M. Wijdicks).

0733-8619/06/$ - see front matter © 2006 Elsevier Inc. All rights reserved.
doi:10.1016/j.ncl.2006.01.005
neurologic.theclinics.com

peripheral causes. The following cases illustrate some of the clinical problems encountered in ICUs.

Case 1

A 50-year-old man is admitted to an ICU after colonic surgery. Postoperatively he remains mechanically ventilated after he develops staphylococcus aureus septicemia, hypotension, liver failure, and renal failure requiring continuous venovenous hemofiltration. He is sedated and paralyzed with neuromuscular blockers (NMBs) to control agitation and improve oxygenation. Four weeks later, sedatives and NMBs are discontinued. By this time he has received a cumulative dose of 500 mg of dexamethasone, 120 mg of atracurium, cyclosporine, fentanyl, lorazepam, and midazolam. Even 3 days after discontinuing NMBs, however, weaning the patient off the ventilator proves difficult. His nurse notices that the patient is unable to move any of his limbs and communicates only by facial expressions. Examination reveals a patient who has complete flaccid quadriplegia, intact sensations, and normal facial expressions. Other cranial nerves are normal. Deep tendon reflexes are absent and plantar reflexes are mute. A serum creatine kinase (CK) level is normal (329 U/L [range, 52–336 U/L]). A brain CT is normal.

Nerve conduction studies show low-amplitude compound muscle action potentials (CMAPs) with normal distal latencies and conduction velocities and sensory nerve action potentials (SNAPs) in all nerves, including the phrenic nerve. Electromyography (EMG) shows scattered fibrillation potentials and small polyphasic rapidly recruited motor unit potentials in proximal muscles. Repetitive nerve stimulation (RNS) studies are normal. Muscle biopsy shows features of a necrotizing myopathy variant of CIM. He fails to improve and expires after another 2 weeks.

Case 2

A 45-year-old man is admitted in a stuporous state to an ICU and immediately is intubated and mechanically ventilated. His sensorium does not improve during 1 week, and he remains ventilator dependent. He develops fever after a day in the ICU. The medical team also notices decreased spontaneous limb movements. All laboratory parameters are normal except for a mild peripheral leukocytosis. Brain CT also is normal. Review of the history reveals that he had been an avid gardener who used to work shirtless in his garden. He recently has complained of many mosquito bites and had flu-like symptoms for a week preceding this admission. Examination reveals a stuporous patient who has flaccid asymmetric weakness (involving predominantly the right arm and left leg) and sluggish reflexes. Lumbar puncture–cerebrospinal fluid (LP-CSF) shows 270 cells with lymphocytic predominance and raised protein levels (75 mg). IgM for West Nile virus (WNV) is positive. Brain MRI shows hyperintense CSF and leptomeningeal enhancement consistent with meningitis. Supportive care is continued, and he recovers after 2 weeks of ICU care.

Evaluation of patients in ICUs who have generalized weakness

These cases illustrate some of the common problems encountered with patients in ICUs. It often is difficult to ascertain the exact time of onset and pattern of weakness, and weakness is detected incidentally or during attempts to wean patients from the ventilator. The initial step to determine is if a central process or peripheral neuromuscular problem is the cause of weakness. This may be complicated by encephalopathy or sedation (resulting from drugs, metabolic processes, sepsis, seizures, or the primary disease process) and intubation. Patients also have many indwelling intravascular catheters or restraints, and a thorough clinical examination often is difficult. Nevertheless, a careful history should be taken, medication charts reviewed, and laboratory tests performed. Common medications interfering with neuromuscular functioning include NMBs, steroids, antiretrovirals [4], statins [5,6], and fibrates.

Clinical examination should concentrate on findings, such as muscle wasting or swelling, muscle tenderness, muscle tone, fasciculations or myokymia, percussion myotonia, tendon reflexes, and skin lesions. Important skin lesions include the heliotrope rash of dermatomyositis (DM), exanthematous rashes associated with viral infections, purpura or petechiae, telangiectasias, digital ulcers or splinter hemorrhages, Janeway's lesions, and Osler's nodes. Fundus examination may reveal Roth's spots or retinal hemorrhages. Subtle twitching of the extremities can betray status epilepticus in patients who are encephalopathic.

A simple mnemonic, MUSCLES, is helpful in recalling some of the common causes of generalized weakness in ICUs (Box 1). Box 2 lists common central and peripheral causes of weakness in ICUs.

An algorithm to guide the clinical approach to these patients is provided in Fig. 1. Other investigations (Box 3) also are helpful in identifying the underlying neurologic disorder.

Spinal cord disorders

Spinal cord injuries are common in patients who have polytrauma and MRI should be considered in these patients. Ischemic myelopathy should be considered in patients who have a history of aortic surgeries or aortic dissections. Several viruses, including coxsackie, echovirus, herpes, Epstein-Barr, and CMV, are associated with infectious myelitis [7]. Antiviral agents should be considered for specific agents—acyclovir, valacyclovir, or famciclovir for herpes myelitis; acyclovir for Epstein-Barr virus myelitis; and ganciclovir or foscarnet for CMV myelitis. Bacterial infections are more likely to result in a parainfectious myelopathy. Sometimes, contiguous spread of infection results in an epidural abscess with development of back pain, fever, or signs of myelopathy. Peripheral leukocytosis and elevation of the erythrocyte sedimentation rate are common accompaniments. Epidural abscess is

---

Box 1. Mnemonic for differential diagnosis of generalized weakness in ICUs

M—medications (steroids, NMBs, zidovudine, amiodarone)
U—undiagnosed neuromuscular disorder (myasthenia gravis, Lambert-Eaton myasthenic syndrome [LEMS], inflammatory myopathies, mitochondrial myopathy, acid maltase deficiency)
S—spinal cord disease (ischemia, compression, trauma, vasculitis, demyelination)
C—CIM, CIP
L—loss of muscle mass (cachectic myopathy, rhabdomyolysis)
E—electrolyte disorders (hypokalemia, hypophosphatemia, hypermagnesemia)
S—systemic illness (porphyria, AIDS, vasculitis, paraneoplastic, toxic)

Modified from Wijdicks EFM. Neurology of critical illness. CNS series. 1st ed. New York: FA Davis; 1995. p. 34–9; with permission.

---

treated with laminectomy and spinal cord decompression and antibiotic therapy.

A spinal epidural hematoma resulting in cord compression is another rare condition that should be kept in mind. MRI is the technique of choice to delineate spinal cord lesions.

Anterior horn cell disorders

Acute poliomyelitis resulting from poliovirus was a leading cause of respiratory failure in the early half of the twentieth century. With its eradication, other viral infections, such as WNV, have taken its place [8]. Severe WNV infection results in a meningoencephalitis and an acute flaccid asymmetric paralysis [9]. The flaccid weakness mimics GBS but is accompanied by fever; encephalopathy; predominantly proximal, asymmetric weakness; electrophysiologic evidence of axonopathy [10]; and CSF evidence of lymphocytic pleocytosis with elevated proteins. ELISA for IgM antibody to WNV is the test of choice and is highly sensitive. MRI shows enhancement of the cauda equina, spinal cord signal changes, and cerebral parenchymal or leptomeningeal signal changes [11]. No specific therapy is available as yet for WNV and treatment mainly is supportive.

Amyotrophic lateral sclerosis sometimes can present with respiratory failure resulting from primary involvement of the phrenic motor neurons [12], although the diagnosis usually is clear-cut on electrophysiologic studies. Other rare anterior horn cell disorders include paraneoplastic motor neuron disorders [13].

Polyneuropathies

Acquired neuropathy in patients who are critically ill was described first by Brown and colleagues under the rubric, CIP [14]. Recent studies show that CIP and its muscle counterpart, CIM, are among the most common disorders resulting in weakness in patients who are in ICUs [2].

Several conditions, including sepsis, systemic inflammatory response syndrome (SIRS), multiorgan dysfunction syndrome, status asthmaticus, and medications, such as NMB agents, corticosteroids, and cytotoxic drugs, are important in the development of these syndromes [15–19]. These conditions are encountered in approximately 30% to 60% of patients who are critically ill and usually are detected approximately 1 week after admission and mechanical ventilation [20,21].

Pulmonary and cardiac causes of failure to wean usually are excluded before neuromuscular weakness is suspected. Typical patients who have CIM/CIP have a flaccid areflexic quadriparesis with sparing of cranial nerves and a variable sensory examination. Nerve conduction studies show low CMAP amplitudes with preservation of SNAP amplitudes in CIM and absent SNAPs in CIP. Phrenic nerve studies and needle EMG of the respiratory muscles also can establish CIM/CIP as the cause of failure to wean from the ventilator. CPK levels are helpful early in the illness in approximately 50% of patients who have CIM.

Muscle biopsy is helpful in subtyping CIM. Four subtypes of CIM have been identified on muscle biopsy—necrotizing, cachectic, acute rhabdomyolysis, and thick filament (myosin) loss type [20,22–24]. Of these, the prognosis is poorest in the necrotizing variant and better in the other variants. Treatment of these syndromes mainly is supportive and rests on aggressive management of the underlying sepsis/SIRS. Intravenous immunoglobulin (IVIg) is not useful in patients who have CIP or CIM [25]. The long-term outcome after CIP is better than that for patients who have CIM [26,27]. Occasionally, diagnostic confusion arises when patients in ICUs are believed to have GBS. The clinical features of GBS, however, are distinct from CIM/CIP. Patients with GBS, in contrast to those patients with CIM or CIP, have weakness prior to ICU admission and have conspicuous cranial nerve involvement, albuminocytologic dissociation, and demyelinating features on nerve conduction studies [14].

In equatorial areas, neurotoxic marine poisoning is another consideration. Acute flaccid paralysis is seen in individuals who consume certain species of fish. The most common poisonings occur from ingestion of pufferfish (Fugu) or certain species of shellfish (mussels, oysters, and clams) [28]. Tetrodotoxin poisoning from Fugu can resemble GBS. Paralysis can occur within 10 minutes after ingestion of pufferfish, and the diagnosis primarily is clinical [29]. Electrophysiologic studies reveal reduced conduction velocities and low sensory and motor amplitudes and may be difficult to differentiate from GBS. Analysis of uneaten fish or patients' urine or serum may

Box 2. Conditions presenting with generalized weakness in ICUs

Muscle diseases
- CIM
- Inflammatory myopathies: PM, DM
- Hypokalemic myopathy
- Rhabdomyolysis
- Muscular dystrophies
- Myotonic dystrophy
- Mitochondrial myopathies
- Acid maltase deficiency

Neuromuscular junction disorders
- Myasthenia gravis
- NMB agent–induced weakness
- Antibiotic-induced myasthenia
- Organophosphorus poisoning
- Snake bite
- Insect toxins
- LEMS
- Congenital myasthenic syndromes
- Hypermagnesemia
- Botulism
- Tick paralysis

Peripheral neuropathies
- Acute inflammatory demyelinating polyneuropathy
- Chronic idiopathic demyelinating polyneuropathy
- CIP
- Phrenic neuropathies
- Toxic neuropathy
- Vasculitis
- Porphyric neuropathy
- Diphtheria
- Lymphoma
- Cytomegalovirus (CMV)-related polyradiculoneuropathy
- Marine toxins (pufferfish, shellfish poisoning)

Anterior horn cell disorders
- Amyotrophic lateral sclerosis
- Paraneoplastic motor neuron disease
- West Nile virus infection
- Acute poliomyelitis
- Spinal muscular atrophy

Spinal cord disorders
- Traumatic spinal cord injury
- Hematoma
- Spinal cord infarction
- Epidural abscess
- Demyelination (MS, Devic's disease, acute disseminated encephalomyelitis [ADEM], transverse myelitis)
- Infective myelitis (coxsackie A,B, CMV, mycoplasma, legionella, herpes)

Intracranial disorders
- Multi-infarct state
- Brainstem infarction or hemorrhage
- Status epilepticus
- Subarachnoid hemorrhage
- ADEM
- Intracerebral hemorrhage
- Hypoxic-ischemic encephalopathy
- Meningeoencephalitis
- Central pontine myelinolysis

detect tetrodotoxin. Early testing is important, as high-performance liquid chromatography in urine samples likely is negative after 5 days. Paralytic shellfish poisoning is similar to tetrodotoxin poisoning. Treatment mainly is supportive and antidotes are not available. Although ciguatera poisoning is better known, it rarely produces generalized weakness.

Other polyneuropathies resulting in weakness in ICUs are rare but include acute vasculitic neuropathies, acute porphyria, drug-induced neuropathies, and the AIDS-associated polyradiculopathies.

Neuromuscular junction disorders

Neuromuscular junction disorders probably are the second most common cause of weakness in ICUs. Common conditions include prolonged neuromuscular blockade, myasthenia gravis, LEMS, and drug-induced or iatrogenic myasthenic syndromes. RNS and assessment of acetylcholine receptor antibody titers are helpful in subtyping the myasthenic syndrome. Iatrogenic or drug-induced myasthenia always should be considered (Box 4). It also must be remembered that all myasthenic patients do not show a uniform response to anticholinesterases. Patients who are seronegative (especially those who are MuSK antibody positive) may even have a poor or hypersensitivity response to anticholinesterase agents [30,31]. These patients may require plasma exchange during their myasthenic crises [32].

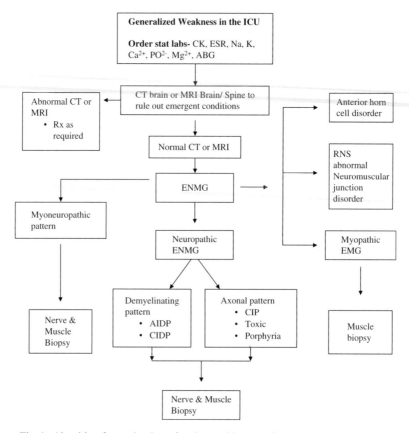

Fig. 1. Algorithm for evaluation of patients with generalized weakness in the ICU.

High-rate RNS studies and anti–VGCC antibodies identify patients who have LEMS. LEMS more often than not is a paraneoplastic syndrome (P-LEMS) that responds variably to 3,4-diaminopyridine or IVIg [33]. Plasma exchange is an alternative in poor responders [34].

Several NMBs are used in patients who are in ICUs to facilitate mechanical ventilation. Any of these NMBs (such as pancuronium, vecuronium, atracurium [35], cisatracurium [36], or doxacurium) can prolong neuromuscular blockade in the presence of metabolic acidosis, electrolyte disturbances, or sepsis.

Less common neuromuscular junction disorders seen in ICUs include botulism, tick paralysis, and hypermagnesemia. Botulism mimics GBS but has additional features of ophthalmoplegia with papillary involvement and autonomic features, such as a dry mouth and paralytic ileus. RNS shows features of a presynaptic neuromuscular junction disorder. Botulinum toxin can be identified in stool, serum, or suspected food samples. Hypermagnesemia is a rare but usually iatrogenic disorder that mimics LEMS. Its similarity with LEMS lies in the fact that magnesium is

---

Box 3. Laboratory investigations in the diagnosis of neuromuscular weakness

Hemogram
Erythrocyte sedimentation rate.
Electrolytes—sodium, potassium, calcium, phosphorus, magnesium, arterial blood gases
Muscle enzymes—CK, serum lactate levels
Autoantibody panel—Anti-Jo1 antibodies, antibodies to the PM-Scl nucleolar antigen complex, acetylcholine receptor antibodies, anti-MuSK antibodies, anti–voltage-gated calcium channel antibodies (VGCC)
Electrophysiologic studies—nerve conduction study(including phrenic nerve study), EMG (including respiratory), diaphragmatic muscles, RNS, single fiber EMG
CSF examination to look for albumino-cytologic dissociation, pleocytosis, malignant cells, or cultures.
CT or MRI of brain and spine with gadolinium
Muscle and nerve biopsy, with overlying skin if possible
Chest radiograph/CT chest to look for contributory parenchymal lung diseases and thymoma and other neoplastic conditions

---

a competitive blocker of calcium at the presynaptic junction, preventing calcium entry into the presynaptic terminal (in LEMS, antibodies against VGCC prevent calcium entry into the presynaptic terminal). Patients develop respiratory failure, generalized weakness, and diminished reflexes [37]. It is seen in patients who have renal failure and who receive magnesium-containing laxatives or antacids or patients who have eclampsia and who are administered magnesium sulfate for seizure control.

Tick paralysis is rare and encountered only in North America and Australia. It mimics GBS with an ascending motor paralysis, preserved sensations, areflexia, and complete ophthalmoplegia. During sucking, the ticks release toxins that block transmitter release from motor nerve terminals. The tick usually is found on the scalp, behind the ear, or in some other moist, warm, hairy area of the body. Removal of the tick is necessary to ameliorate neuromuscular block. Tick removal rapidly reverses American tick paralysis. Australian tick paralysis can worsen for a few more days before clinical improvement is seen [29].

Myopathies

The most common myopathy encountered in patients in ICUs probably is CIM. As it is discussed previously with CIP, further mention is omitted from this section. Among acquired myopathies, inflammatory myopathies

---

Box 4. Partial list of drugs that can worsen neuromuscular function

D-penicillamine
Interferon-α
Aminoglycosides
Magnesium-containing laxatives, antacids
NMBs
Quinolones
Polymyxin antibiotics
Quinidine, quinine
β-blockers
Calcium channel blockers
Phenytoin
Corticosteroids
Lithium
Chloroquine

---

are among the most common types encountered in ICUs—DM and polymyositis (PM). DM is easy to recognize by virtue of its accompanying skin rash. The rash is erythematous, periorbital, and purplish and can be accompanied by rashes over the knuckles (Gottron's sign) or subcutaneous calcifications. CK levels often are elevated. Electrophysiologic studies (electromyography) and muscle biopsy help in establishing the diagnosis. Autoantibodies have only a limited clinical relevance in the management of these conditions. Corticosteroids are the mainstay of therapy for patients who have inflammatory myopathies, although patients who have respiratory failure in ICUs may benefit from with IV methylprednisolone [38]. Steroid-sparing agents, such as methotrexate or azathioprine, often are considered as soon as the diagnosis is made [39,40]. IVIg has a limited role and is used only as a second-line agent in DM when the disease fails to respond to steroids [41,42].

Electrolyte disturbances rarely result in severe weakness in ICUs. The exception is hypokalemia, which can be acquired [43] or familial Hypokalemic periodic paralysis, resulting from familial periodic paralysis or thyrotoxic periodic paralysis, presents with recurrent weakness and infrequently with respiratory failure [44].

Rhabdomyolysis often presents with focal rather than generalized weakness. This entity should be considered in the presence of arterial occlusion, compartment syndromes, or trauma. It often presents with swollen, tender muscles, focal weakness, and elevated CK levels (> 10,000 IU). Nevertheless, subclinical rhabdomyolysis can coexist with generalized weakness in one of the subtypes of CIM. Iatrogenic rhabdomyolysis resulting from medications, such as statins, fibrates, colchicine, or zidovudine, should be ruled out.

Intracranial disorders

Although neuromuscular causes account for the majority of patients who have generalized weakness, intracranial conditions always should be considered. Posterior circulation strokes (especially pontine infarctions) can result in a locked-in state, where patients are able to communicate only via eye blinks. Multiple strokes can be seen in patients who have underlying infective endocarditis or have undergone cardiac surgery. Depending on the type of cardiac surgery, the frequency of strokes may vary from 2% to 7% [45]. Rarely, previously unrecognized brainstem tumor or lesions can present in the postoperative phase with difficulty in weaning from the ventilator or generalized weakness.

Critically ill patients often are malnourished and predisposed to changes in electrolyte and fluid balances. In this setting, individuals who are alcoholic, have suffered extensive burns, or have undergone liver transplantation are especially prone to developing central pontine myelinolysis or extra pontine myelinolysis. This can present with a locked-in state or deterioration in sensorium and seizures [46,47].

Summary

The differential diagnosis of generalized weakness in ICU patients is quite broad. Although neuromuscular disorders are the most common causes of generalized weakness, a thorough evaluation is necessary to delineate the underlying cause of weakness. Biochemical studies, neuroimaging, and electrophysiologic studies help to delineate most of the common disorders associated with weakness. Prompt identification of a neurologic disorder and initiation of therapy speeds up recovery and reduces morbidity and mortality in these patients.

References

[1] Rudis MI, Guslits BJ, Peterson EL, et al. Economic impact of prolonged motor weakness complicating neuromuscular blockade in the intensive care unit. Crit Care Med 1996;24: 1749–56.

[2] Lacomis D, Petrella JT, Giuliani MJ. Causes of neuromuscular weakness in the intensive care unit: a study of ninety-two patients. Muscle Nerve 1998;21:610–7.

[3] Bleck TP, Smith MC, Pierre-Louis SJ, et al. Neurologic complications of critical medical illnesses. Crit Care Med 1993;21:98–103.

[4] Dalakas MC. Peripheral neuropathy and antiretroviral drugs. J Peripher Nerv Syst 2001;6: 14–20.

[5] Bae J, Jarcho JA, Denton MD, et al. Statin specific toxicity in organ transplant recipients: case report and review of the literature. J Nephrol 2002;15:317–9.

[6] Ravnan SL, Locke C, Yee WP, et al. Cerivastatin-induced rhabdomyolysis: 11 case reports. Pharmacotherapy 2002;22:533–7.
[7] Berger JR, Sabet A. Infectious myelopathies. Semin Neurol 2002;22:133–42.
[8] Bouffard JP, Riudavets MA, Holman R, et al. Neuropathology of the brain and spinal cord in human West Nile virus infection. Clin Neuropathol 2004;23:59–61.
[9] Sejvar JJ, Leis AA, Stokic DS, et al. Acute flaccid paralysis and West Nile virus infection. Emerg Infect Dis 2003;9:788–93.
[10] Flaherty ML, Wijdicks EF, Stevens JC, et al. Clinical and electrophysiologic patterns of flaccid paralysis due to West Nile virus. Mayo Clin Proc 2003;78:1245–8.
[11] Jeha LE, Sila CA, Lederman RJ, et al. West Nile virus infection: a new acute paralytic illness. Neurology 2003;61:55–9.
[12] Chen R, Grand'Maison F, Strong MJ, et al. Motor neuron disease presenting as acute respiratory failure: a clinical and pathological study. J Neurol Neurosurg Psychiatry 1996;60:455–8.
[13] Forman D, Rae-Grant AD, Matchett SC, et al. A reversible cause of hypercapnic respiratory failure: lower motor neuronopathy associated with renal cell carcinoma. Chest 1999;115:899–901.
[14] Bolton CF, Laverty DA, Brown JD, et al. Critically ill polyneuropathy: electrophysiological studies and differentiation from Guillain-Barre syndrome. J Neurol Neurosurg Psychiatry 1986;49:563–73.
[15] Perea M, Picon M, Miro O, et al. Acute quadriplegic myopathy with loss of thick (myosin) filaments following heart transplantation. J Heart Lung Transplant 2001;20:1136–41.
[16] Wijdicks EF, Litchy WJ, Wiesner RH, et al. Neuromuscular complications associated with liver transplantation. Muscle Nerve 1996;19:696–700.
[17] Ghaus N, Bohlega S, Rezeig M. Neurological complications in liver transplantation. J Neurol 2001;248:1042–8.
[18] Miro O, Salmeron JM, Masanes F, et al. Acute quadriplegic myopathy with myosin-deficient muscle fibres after liver transplantation: defining the clinical picture and delimiting the risk factors. Transplantation 1999;67:1144–51.
[19] Cassidy JV, Bolton DT, Haynes SR, et al. Acute rhabdomyolysis after cardiac transplantation: a diagnostic conundrum. Paediatr Anaesth 2002;12:729–32.
[20] Bolton CF. Neuromuscular manifestations of critical illness. Muscle Nerve 2005;32:140–63.
[21] Tennila A, Salmi T, Pettila V, et al. Early signs of critical illness polyneuropathy in ICU patients with systemic inflammatory response syndrome or sepsis. Intensive Care Med 2000;26:1360–3.
[22] Bolton CF. Sepsis and the systemic inflammatory response syndrome: neuromuscular manifestations. Crit Care Med 1996;24:1408–16.
[23] Hund E. Neurological complications of sepsis: critical illness polyneuropathy and myopathy. J Neurol 2001;248:929–34.
[24] Sander HW, Golden M, Danon MJ. Quadriplegic areflexic ICU illness: selective thick filament loss and normal nerve histology. Muscle Nerve 2002;26:499–505.
[25] Wijdicks EF, Fulgham JR. Failure of high dose intravenous immunoglobulins to alter the clinical course of critical illness polyneuropathy. Muscle Nerve 1994;17:1494–5.
[26] Fletcher SN, Kennedy DD, Ghosh IR, et al. Persistent neuromuscular and neurophysiologic abnormalities in long-term survivors of prolonged critical illness. Crit Care Med 2003;31:1012–6.
[27] Hund EF, Fogel W, Krieger D, et al. Critical illness polyneuropathy: clinical findings and outcomes of a frequent cause of neuromuscular weaning failure. Crit Care Med 1996;24:1328–33.
[28] Isbister GK, Kiernan MC. Neurotoxic marine poisoning. Lancet Neurol 2005;4:219–28.
[29] Harris JB, Goonetilleke A. Animal poisons and the nervous system: what the neurologist needs to know. J Neurol Neurosurg Psychiatry 2004;75(Suppl 3):iii40–6.

[30] Liyanage Y, Hoch W, Beeson D, et al. The agrin/muscle-specific kinase pathway: new targets for autoimmune and genetic disorders at the neuromuscular junction. Muscle Nerve 2002;25: 4–16.

[31] Lavrnic D, Losen M, Vujic A, et al. The features of myasthenia gravis with autoantibodies to MuSK. J Neurol Neurosurg Psychiatry 2005;76:1099–102.

[32] Sanders DB, El-Salem K, Massey JM, et al. Clinical aspects of MuSK antibody positive seronegative MG. Neurology 2003;60:1978–80.

[33] Maddison P, Newsom-Davis J. Treatment for Lambert-Eaton myasthenic syndrome. Cochrane Database Syst Rev 2005;18:CD003279.

[34] Newsom-Davis J. Therapy in myasthenia gravis and Lambert-Eaton myasthenic syndrome. Semin Neurol 2003;23:191–8.

[35] Hoey LL, Joslin SM, Nahum A, et al. Prolonged neuromuscular blockade in two critically ill patients treated with atracurium. Pharmacotherapy 1995;15:254–9.

[36] Davis NA, Rodgers JE, Gonzalez ER, et al. Prolonged weakness after cisatracurium infusion: a case report. Crit Care Med 1998;26:1290–2.

[37] Krendel DA. Hypermagnesemia and neuromuscular transmission. Semin Neurol 1990;10: 42–5.

[38] Matsubara S, Sawa Y, Takamori M, et al. Pulsed intravenous methylprednisolone combined with oral steroids as the initial treatment of inflammatory myopathies. J Neurol Neurosurg Psychiatry 1994;57:1008.

[39] Mastaglia F, Phillips B, Zilko P, et al. Relapses in idiopathic inflammatory myopathies. Muscle Nerve 1999;22:1160–1.

[40] Miro O, Laguna M, Grau JM. Relapses in idiopathic inflammatory myopathies. Muscle Nerve 1999;22:1159–60.

[41] Dalakas MC, Illa I, Dambrosia JM, et al. A controlled trial of high-dose intravenous immune globulin infusions as treatment for dermatomyositis. N Engl J Med 1993;329: 1993–2000.

[42] Dalakas MC. Intravenous immunoglobulin in autoimmune neuromuscular diseases. JAMA 2004;291:2367–75.

[43] Chhabra A, Patwari AK, Aneja S, et al. Neuromuscular manifestations of diarrhea related hypokalemia. Indian Pediatr 1995;32:409–15.

[44] Liu YC, Tsai WS, Chau T, et al. Acute hypercapnic respiratory failure due to thyrotoxic periodic paralysis. Am J Med Sci 2004;327:264–7.

[45] Boeken U, Litmathe J, Feindt P, et al. Neurological complications after cardiac surgery: risk factors and correlation to the surgical procedure. Thorac Cardiovasc Surg 2005;53:33–6.

[46] Martin RJ. Central pontine and extrapontine myelinolysis: the osmotic demyelination syndromes. J Neurol Neurosurg Psychiatry 2004;75(Suppl 3):iii22–8.

[47] Ashrafian H, Davey P. A review of the causes of central pontine myelinosis: yet another apoptotic illness? Eur J Neurol 2001;8:103–9.

NEUROLOGIC
CLINICS

Neurol Clin 24 (2006) 385–403

Functional Symptoms in Neurology: Case Studies

Jon Stone, MB, ChB, MRCP*, Michael Sharpe, MD, FRCP, FRCPsych

School of Molecular and Clinical Medicine, University of Edinburgh, Western General Hospital, Crewe Road, Edinburgh EH4 2XU, Scotland

Approximately one third of new patients presenting to a neurologist have symptoms such as pain, fatigue, numbness, weakness, blackouts, and dizziness, which are either not explained by disease or only partially explained by disease. For many neurologists, patients with these symptoms are frustrating to manage. Although medical students are taught that many of these symptoms have a psychological basis, this is usually the last thing a patient wishes to hear.

In this article, the authors discuss five patients presenting with various symptoms that are unexplained by recognized neurological disease. These are referred to as functional symptoms, but they might also be called conversion symptoms, psychogenic, dissociative, nonorganic, somatoform or hysterical symptoms. Special attention is given to the motor and sensory symptoms most likely to find their way into a neurologic clinic.

Using these case studies, the authors hope to highlight practical clinical issues in the diagnosis and management of functional symptoms. The case reports have been adapted and anonymized from experiences with real patients. A comprehensive standard review of the diagnosis and management of functional symptoms can be found elsewhere [1,2].

Case 1: Blackouts

A 33–year old mother of three is referred because of increasingly frequent blackouts over the previous 3 months. Her initial description of the events is noticeably lacking in detail. She says that she has no warning and simply

---

* Corresponding author.
E-mail address: Jon.Stone@ed.ac.uk (J. Stone).

0733-8619/06/$ - see front matter © 2006 Elsevier Inc. All rights reserved.
doi:10.1016/j.ncl.2006.01.008

comes round on the floor feeling tired and disoriented. On one occasion she said she had bitten the tip of her tongue and on two others had been incontinent of urine. A family member who was a care worker with learning disabled people labeled it an epileptic fit. The witness described a gradual build up of hyperventilation over 5 minutes with increasing distress followed by a "shaking attack" lasting approximately 5 minutes. The witness also described in the patient a lack of a tonic phase, closed eyes and mouth, and a period of crying that commonly followed the episode. The patient has no memory of this and is surprised to hear the description.

Further questioning reveals that the patient also has episodes when she feels generally "spaced out," lasting 10 minutes or so when she can hear what is going on around her but cannot respond. Witnesses say that during these episodes she looks tired but has no automatisms. She admits that over the past few months she has felt generally tired, with hypersomnia and irritability, and has been dropping things. There is a past medical history of hysterectomy at the age of 26 because of heavy and painful periods, and a history of negative investigation for a whispering dysphonia and chronic low back pain. There is also a history of previous assault with a head injury, and the patient wonders if this is relevant. She says that she is frightened about her attacks but is keen to point out that she is not stressed or depressed. Physical examination is normal. She would like to start medication to prevent epilepsy, which was the diagnosis made by two previous doctors.

What Is the Diagnosis and How Are You Going to Confirm It?

The primary differential diagnosis of blackouts is commonly epilepsy, syncope, or nonepileptic attacks/pseudoseizures. Table 1 lists clinical features, including those relevant to this case, which should guide decision making. For a full review, the interested reader is referred elsewhere [3,4].

None of the features listed in Table 1 make the diagnosis in isolation, but in this case, the history and description of the attacks taken together suggests a diagnosis of nonepileptic attacks or pseudoseizures. The patient has a history of functional dysphonia and has had a hysterectomy for nonpathological reasons at a young age. The attacks as described would be unusually long for generalized tonic-clonic seizures, which normally last no longer than 90 seconds. The presence of closed eyes during a shaking attack is particularly suggestive, as is weeping or an emotional outburst after the event. Tongue biting, incontinence, and injury can all occur in nonepileptic attacks, although some authors have reported that lateral tongue biting is specific for epilepsy.

Clinical suspicions should be verified whenever possible, particularly in a difficult case such as this, by EEG recording of the attack itself with accompanying video recording of concurrent behavior. Many patients have spontaneous attacks during a routine EEG. The chance of this occurring can be increased by adding physiologic induction techniques such as hyperventilation and photic stimulation. There is also evidence that sympathetic

Table 1
Clinical indicators of nonepileptic attacks compared with epilepsy and syncope

Clinical indicator	Nonepileptic attacks	Epilepsy	Syncope
Useful			
Eyelids/mouth	Often shut with resistance to eye opening	Often open	Often open
Duration of attack	Often >2 min	Rarely >2 min	Rarely >1 min
Onset	Often >2 min	Usually rapid (although temporal lobe seizures may be longer)	Rapid
Postictal weeping	Common	Rare	Rare
Limb movement	Asynchronous; ↔ semipurposeful; maintaining rhythmicity	Synchronous, rarely interacting with environment (in a tonic clonic seizure). Decreasing frequency	Stiffening or myoclonic jerks lasting up to 30 s is common
Tongue-biting	Tip (occasional) Side (rare)	Side (common) Tip (rare)	Tip (occasional) Side (rare)
Opisthotonus/ arched back	Occasional	Rare	Rare
Purposeful movements	Occasional	Rare	Rare
Side-to-side head shaking	Common	Rare	Rare
Responsiveness to touch	Occasional	Rare	Rare
Prolonged atonia	Common	Rare	Rare
History of multiple functional symptoms/ multiple surgery	Common	Occasional	Occasional
Less useful/not useful			
Urinary incontinence	Occasional	Common	Occasional
Injury	Common	Common	Common
Aura	Common	Common	Common

Adapted from Reuber M, Elger CE. Psychogenic nonepileptic seizures: a review and update. Epilepsy Behav 2003;4:205–16; with permission.

and transparent verbal suggestion may precipitate attacks [5]. If video EEG is not available, then home video may also be useful. Measurement of serum prolactin has been advocated as a useful test for seizures as it is often raised 10–20 minutes after a generalized or complex partial seizure [6]. However, it may also be elevated after syncope [7], and sometimes after nonepileptic seizures [8]. It requires a baseline value, and in practice it is often performed at the wrong time. Induction of seizures using saline and placebo has also been described. This may be justified on rare occasions when reversing a potentially dangerous diagnosis of epilepsy but may harm the doctor-patient relationship and be viewed as unethical if not planned and used with care [3].

Once You Have Secured the Diagnosis, How Are You Going to Explain It to the Patient?

Two common approaches to this problem are (a) to tackle the problem as a psychological one right from the outset even if this is not what the patient wishes to hear or (b) to use a more physiological explanation initially (describing the process of dissociation in terms of a trance or a short circuit of the nervous system) and introduce psychological aspects later. The best approach is uncertain. Patients with nonepileptic attacks often believe strongly they are suffering from a disease process and not a psychiatric illness [9]. The first approach may be less acceptable initially but may produce acceptance of subsequent psychological treatments. This dilemma is reflected in the numerous terms for nonepileptic attacks, which range from functional seizures or nonepileptic attacks, which patients do not find immediately offensive, to more overtly psychological terms, such as psychogenic seizures [10].

Despite the uncertainty over labels, it seems likely that the term used and the explanation given is probably less important than the doctor's ability to convey the message that (a) they believe the patient's description of symptoms, (b) they do not think the attacks are "faked" or their fault, and (c) they are willing to help. It is therefore important to use the explanation you feel most comfortable with. There is some preliminary evidence that anger at the diagnosis relates to poor outcome [11], although this requires further testing. Table 2 provides elements of an explanation of functional symptoms that the authors find helpful.

Once an explanation has been given, the neurologist's role in treating nonepileptic seizures may include simple advice about detecting and managing warning signs of attacks, such as panic symptoms or dissociation; clear advice to family members about what to do during an attack; withdrawal of anticonvulsant drugs if already started [12]; follow-up to ensure that the diagnosis is accepted; and onward referral for psychiatric assessment. Some patients with nonepileptic attacks improve with simple measures; others require more prolonged treatment, including treatment of any comorbid emotional disorders with antidepressants or psychotherapy [13]. As with epilepsy, there are patients with treatment-resistant attacks who require containment strategies to avoid harm and repeated admission to a hospital. There are currently no randomized trials to guide practice, although therapies such as cognitive behavioral therapy appear useful in a range of other symptoms unexplained by disease [14] and show promise in nonepileptic attacks [15].

Table 2
Elements of a constructive explanation of functional neurologic symptoms

Element	Example
1. Indicate that you believe the patient.	"I do not think you are making up or imagining your symptoms."
2. Explain what the patient does *not* have.	"You do not have MS, epilepsy, etc."
3. Explain what the patient *does* have.	"You have functional weakness. This is a common problem. Your nervous system is not damaged but it is not working properly. That is why you cannot move your arm."
4. Emphasize that the condition is common.	"I see lots of patients with similar symptoms."
5. Emphasize reversibility.	"Because there is no damage, you have the potential to get better."
6. Emphasize that self-help is a key part of getting better.	"I know you didn't bring this on but there are things you can do to help it get better."
7. Metaphors may be useful.	"The hardware is alright, but there is a software problem," "It is like a car/piano that's out of tune," "It is like a short-circuit of the nervous system" (nonepileptic attacks).
8. Introduce the role of depression/anxiety.	"If you have been feeling low/worried, that will tend to make the symptoms even worse."
9. Use written information.	Send the patient a clinic letter. Give them a leaflet.
10. Suggest antidepressants.	"We find that so-called antidepressants often help these symptoms even in patients who are not feeling depressed. They are not addictive."
11. Make a psychiatric referral.	"I don't think you're mad, but Dr. X has a lot of experience and interest in helping people like you to manage and overcome their symptoms."

Case 2: Weakness

A 39-year-old man presents to an emergency service having developed left-sided weakness while exercising during physiotherapy. The therapist stated that the patient complained of marked back pain during the session and then collapsed to the ground in agony. He was observed to shake all over for several minutes and appeared to be hyperventilating. When he stopped shaking, he moaned and appeared distant. On coming round, he could not move or feel his left leg and had to be taken by stretcher to the emergency department. He complains of memory loss lasting approximately 30 minutes for the event in the physiotherapy room.

There is a past medical history of chronic back pain with no associated structural abnormality on MRI. He has also been seen in a gastrointestinal clinic on several occasions with nonulcer dyspepsia. Systemic inquiry finds a long history of exhaustion with poor sleep, mental slowing, irritability, and loss of pleasure in life, especially since being medically retired from his work in an office. Like case 1, he looked unhappy but became angry when another doctor suggested his problems may be psychogenic. All investigations, including MRI brain, lumbar puncture, and EEG were normal.

How Are You Going to Look for a Diagnosis of Possible Functional Weakness?

The history alone cannot provide a diagnosis of functional weakness. The differential diagnosis with this history is wide and includes stroke and epilepsy (with Todd's palsy). However, there are several clues to functional weakness in the history given. He has a history of other symptoms not explained by disease, there is a background history of somatic symptoms of depression, and he may have had dissociative amnesia for the onset of the symptoms.

Neuroimaging (preferably MRI with stroke sequences) was warranted in this case, as in most cases of functional weakness. However, normal imaging is insufficient to make the diagnosis, which must rest primarily on the presence of positive findings in the examination. The key finding is inconsistency. For example, there may be virtually no movement on the bed, but walking will demonstrate much more significant ability. The most useful way of looking for inconsistency in patients with leg weakness is to use Hoover's sign (Fig. 1) [16]. For this test, devised by Charles Hoover in 1908, first examine hip extension in the affected leg. This is often selectively weak, which in itself is rather unusual for organic disease. If it is weak, then keep your hand under the heel of the affected leg while testing hip flexion in the normal leg against resistance. If, during this maneuver, hip extension comes back dramatically to normal, Hoover's sign is positive. The test can be performed the other way round by testing for hip extension in the good leg during attempted hip flexion of the affected one, although this is a more difficult sign to interpret. A similar test using hip abduction is also described [17]. Like all physical signs, Hoover's sign is not perfect. It can be falsely positive when patients have cortical neglect or pain. It also does not exclude the presence of comorbid disease and does not differentiate conversion weakness from malingered weakness (no physical test does). However, there is some evidence of its validity, and it is a test that can be repeated. It can also be shown to the patient in a sympathetic manner to convince them of the diagnosis.

Some patients with functional leg weakness will also have a typical dragging monoplegic gait, first described in 1854 by Todd [18] and photographed by Charcot (Fig. 2) [19]. Usually, either the hip is externally or internally rotated to allow the whole leg to drag behind as a single unit. When marked, this is a characteristic sign of the condition.

Collapsing weakness is often mentioned as a sign of functional weakness. Though it is common in functional weakness, it also occurs in patients with neurological disease, particularly when there is pain or neglect [20]. If you

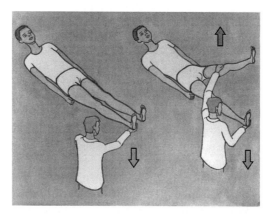

Fig. 1. Hoover's test for functional weakness. This test relies on the patient having weakness of hip extension which then returns to normal when hip flexion against resistance is tested in the opposite leg. (*From* Stone J, Zeman A, Sharpe M. Functional weakness and sensory disturbance. J Neurol Neurosurg Psychiatry 2002;73(3):242).

find collapsing weakness, it can be characterized further by asking the patient to put all their effort into a single push (eg, "At the count of three, stop me from pushing down") or by gradually increasing your resistant force from barely perceptible up to normal over a 5-second period (instead of all at once).

What Is the Risk of Misdiagnosis Using Clinical Examination Like This?

Something that causes a lot of concern, especially to psychiatric colleagues, is the possibility that patients presenting like the one above will

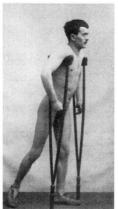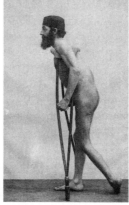

Fig. 2. Dragging monoplegic gait seen in some patients with functional weakness (*From* Charcot J-M. Nouvelle Iconographie de Salpêtrière. Clinique des maladies du systeme nerveux. Publiée sous la direction du par Paul Richer, Gilles de la Tourette, Albert Londe. Paris: Lecrosnier et Babé; 1888).

eventually turn out to have a disease that explains their original presentation. This concern is based, in part, on reports published in the 1960s suggesting a high misdiagnosis rate [21]. Patients themselves are often convinced that there must be a disease to explain their symptoms, especially if they are presented with an alternative psychiatric diagnosis, which they may view as an accusation of malingering.

A recent systematic review of the misdiagnosis of a range of conversion symptoms, including weakness, nonepileptic attacks, and visual symptoms, has questioned this assumption. It found that in 27 published studies the rate of new disease diagnoses emerging at an average of 5 years after the initial diagnosis has, on average, been lower than 5% since 1970, well before CT scanning was widely available [22]. This is comparable with misdiagnosis rates in other neurological and psychiatric diagnoses. Features that may lead the unwary into a misdiagnosis include the presence of an extensive psychiatric history, bizarre symptoms, and gait disorder. Misdiagnosis can also be minimized by being prepared to make two diagnoses—one of a disease diagnosis (such as multiple sclerosis) and the other a functional one (such as additional functional weakness).

What Should I Do If I Think the Patient Needs Psychiatric Management but the Patient Will Not Accept This?

Initial explanation and management of patients with functional weakness can follow similar lines to that described with nonepileptic attacks (case 1). It cannot be overemphasized how important it is to make the patient feel that they are believed. For patients with functional weakness, psychological explanations are particularly unpalatable as the symptom is usually there all the time and it is much harder for them to accept that something psychological could be causing it. The advantage of the term functional weakness is that it allows a transparent discussion about the mechanism of the weakness without having to discuss etiology, which is likely to be complex and vary from patient to patient. For example, it can be explained to the patient that their nervous system is not damaged but is not functioning properly and that this is therefore potentially reversible. Using analogies such as "This is a software problem rather than a hardware problem" can be helpful. Explaining how common it is or using written information will also show to the patient that they have an illness you recognize and can help. The danger is that the patient will interpret this explanation wrongly as having an irreversible neurological disorder that they have no power to influence through their own actions.

Once a patient feels believed, they are much more likely to accept discussion and treatment of psychological aspects of their illness. Preferably, patients should be referred to psychiatrists who are experienced and interested in this problem (such as consultation-liaison psychiatrists or neuropsychiatrists). This is because psychiatrists unfamiliar with this type of work may not pick up emotional disorder in patients who are defensive about the possibility of psychiatric illness and who focus on somatic symptoms. The neurologist making the referral can explain that the psychiatrist is an expert in their condition and can give advice and treatment for managing and overcoming physical and emotional symptoms. It is important for the neurologist to continue to see the patient until the patient has (a) improved, (b) successfully engaged in treatment from a therapist, or (c) failed treatment. Always consider referring a patient with functional weakness for physiotherapy. If the therapist is familiar with the condition, they can reinforce helpful behaviors.

Case 3: A Clenched Fist

A 36-year-old woman presents with a 2-month history of a progressively worsening fixed flexed posture of her right wrist and fingers, which looks as if she is clenching her fist (see Fig. 3 for a similar patient). She recalls that she first noticed it after she sprained her wrist while trying to control one of her children. A wrist radiograph was normal. She was given an elasticized wrist support for a week by her primary care physician. Her pain got worse however and spread up her arm. She started to develop variable numbness and shooting pains in the arm and found that she was using it less than previously. The clenched fist gradually developed over a 2-week period early after the injury. She reported being unable to relax the fingers and was concerned that her fingernails, which she had not been able to cut, were digging into her palm.

Her past medical history was long and included hysterectomy at the age of 26 for painful and heavy bleeding with recurrent abdominal pain since then. She had had numerous laparoscopic divisions of abdominal adhesions and frequent admissions to the gastroenterology ward where she was often given opiates. She also had a history of recurrent blackouts, one of which

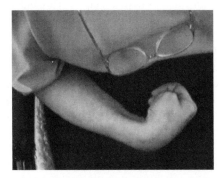

Fig. 3. A clenched fist or fixed dystonia from Schrag's cases series [23]. A proportion of these patients can be demonstrated to be functional. (*From* Schrag A, Trimble M, Quinn N, et al. The syndrome of fixed dystonia: an evaluation of 103 patients. Brain 2004;127(Pt 10):2366; with permission.)

led to intubation and ventilation for presumed status epilepticus but that turned out to be a nonepileptic attack. Previous psychiatric assessments found a history of childhood and adult sexual abuse as well as recurrent episodes of major depression and panic with agoraphobia. One letter suggested that she may have somatization disorder, but this was not something that had apparently been taken notice of by other physicians and surgeons involved with her care.

Examination demonstrated a fixed clenched fist on the right with a 70-degree flexion deformity of the wrist. The patient also tended to flex the right elbow. There was evidence of some collapsing weakness of the right arm, but this was difficult to assess because of pain in the whole arm. There was a mild degree of weakness in the right leg on examination with a positive Hoover's sign, even though the patient did not complain of this.

What Is the Diagnosis? Is the Wrist Sprain Relevant? Is This an Organic or Nonorganic Disorder?

The clenched fist and the inverted ankle are the two most common presentations of fixed dystonia. This is probably an end point of a heterogenous group of disorders, the nature of which has recently been enlightened by a large case series of 103 patients described by Schrag et al [23]. Of the 41 patients in this series that were investigated prospectively, 36% had documented or clinically established psychogenic dystonia according to Fahn and William's criteria [24]. In these criteria, "documented" equates to "persistent relief by psychotherapy, suggestion or placebo, or observed without the movement disorder when 'unobserved.'" Clinically established refers to psychogenic dystonia which is "incongruent with classical dystonia or inconsistent plus other psychogenic signs, multiple somatizations or obvious psychiatric disturbance." Ten percent of patients had no evidence of a psychogenic disorder. These criteria are hard to operationalize but they at least grade the level of uncertainty. Features said to be helpful in making a diagnosis of fixed dystonia include the distribution, a history of sudden onset, a history of physical trauma, the lack of characteristic features such as sensory tricks (geste antagoniste), and the absence of overflow dystonia. Table 3 shows some helpful clinical features in functional dystonia and other functional movement disorders. There are helpful review articles [25,26] and a recent book on this subject [27].

Schrag et al also found a rate of somatization disorder of 29% in this group of patients—with important evidence often found only in primary care records [23]. The gender ratio and psychiatric comorbidity were similar to patients with other somatoform disorders. Physical injury at onset (68%), as in this case, and immobilization in a plaster cast (15%) were identified as important risk factors for developing this symptom.

Is the clenched fist always a functional/nonorganic problem? It seems likely that the proportion of patients in whom this is the case is higher

Table 3
Features and investigations to consider when suspecting a functional or psychogenic movement disorder

	Positive features	Notes
General features	Abrupt onset +/− trauma Variability in frequency, distribution Selective disability	Worsening with anxiety/stress is not specific and occurs with all movement disorders. Many organic movement disorders appear odd, and this should not be a criterion either.
	Dramatic resolution with placebo, suggestion, distraction or after anaesthesia	To look for distraction, ask the patient to carry out a complex motor or cognitive task.
Tremor	The presence of entrainment Worsening when limb is held or weight is placed on it Typical pattern of co-contraction of agonists and antagonists	To look for entrainment in a patient with unilateral tremor, ask the patient to attempt 3Hz rhythmical movement of the normal hand. Look for entrainment of the affected side to the rhythm, or an inability to carry out the instruction.
Dystonia	Inverted ankle or clenched fist onset in an adult	Look for absence of normal features of dystonia (eg, the presence of a geste or overflow dystonia).
	Usually fixed	
Parkinsonism	Reduced tone with synkinesis	Consider carrying out a radiolabeled scan of dopaminergic function (eg., [123I]FP-CIT single-photon emission computed tomography [SPECT]).
Myoclonus	Same as for general features	Consider seeking specialized EEG analysis to look for the presence of a Bereitschaftpotential—not normally seen in typical myoclonus.

than previously recognized, particularly because examination under sedation is required to confirm the diagnosis. However, it is also important to keep an open mind about this symptom, which illustrates well the error of trying to identify a symptom as being organic or nonorganic. It is likely that a complex mixture of biological, physiological, behavioral, psychological, and social factors account for these symptoms (and probably most functional symptoms). There may also be some types of organic disease, such as stiff person syndrome and antibasal ganglia antibody-mediated disease [28], which particularly predispose to fluctuating or psychogenic types of presentation. There is a often overlap with complex regional pain type 1/ reflex sympathetic dystrophy in which similar fixed postures are described [29]. Much of the debate in the literature results from patients and doctors trying to separate out genuine organic disease from nongenuine functional symptoms. If organic and functional problems were considered equally genuine, this would be a step forward in this area.

What Is the Management?

If the problem is intractable, and particularly if the palm is starting to be macerated, it may be helpful diagnostically and therapeutically to examine the patient under sedation, anesthesia, or hypnosis. This allows assessment for the presence of contractures. In addition, such a procedure, if handled well, can be therapeutic in allowing the patient to see that recovery is possible. It may be helpful to record the session on video to show the patient and reinforce your argument for the potential reversibility of the problem.

The reported prognosis for psychogenic movement disorder is gloomy [27]. However, careful explanation, treatment of comorbid psychiatric disorders, and multidisciplinary management along the lines described previously for patients with weakness is likely to offer the best chance of a successful outcome.

Case 4: Unilateral Numbness with a Feeling of Detachment

A 45-year-old woman presents with a 2-year history of numbness and intermittent pain on her right side. She cannot date the onset but the problem seems to have got slowly worse over time. She describes the right side as "heavy," "strange," "as if it doesn't belong to me at times." She is aware that the symptom is variable and sometimes not there at all. When the symptom is intense, she says it feels as if she is "cut in half". At other times she experiences pain in her right knee and hip. Occasionally she feels as if she cannot see or hear properly on the right side either. She reports a continual feeling of exhaustion with insomnia and impaired concentration. On direct questioning she reported frequently feeling detached from her surroundings. This feeling was frightening to her, but she reported feeling reluctant to discuss it with others. She denies feeling depressed but admits that her symptoms have progressed to the point that she is hardly able to enjoy anything. Examination reveals normal power and deep tendon reflexes with a right hemisensory disturbance to light touch, pinprick, and vibration sense in her face, arm, trunk and leg. She has lost the ticklishness of her right foot. Investigations, including MRI brain and spine, neurophysiology, and lumbar puncture, are normal.

What Is the Diagnosis?

This patient has functional hemisensory symptoms, also referred to as hemisensory syndrome. This is one of the most common but least researched functional symptoms [30]. It can be found in many scenarios; for example, it is recognized in patients with chronic generalized pain and in patients with complex regional pain. Most patients with functional weakness also complain of numbness with similar clinical characteristics. It may also present as a primary symptom and was well described by many authors in the late nineteenth and early twentieth centuries (Fig. 4). In the fifteenth to seventeenth centuries, women who were said to be witches because of areas of sensory disturbance may have had this symptom. Patients with hemisensory symptoms such as this frequently complain of blurred vision on the same side (asthenopia) and may be found to have a tubular field defect or spiral visual fields on this side (Figs. 5 and 6). Hearing on the affected side may be perceived to be impaired as well (asthenacusis). For a review of the many tests available to examine functional visual symptoms, the reader is referred elsewhere [31].

Patients with this presentation require a diagnostic work-up if the patient wishes a disease cause to be excluded. Less weight can be placed on the physical signs accompanying functional sensory symptoms than those for functional weakness. These signs include midline splitting (in which the patient has numbness that stops abruptly in the midline rather than 1 to 2 cm lateral to it) and midline splitting of vibration sense (in which the patient feels a tuning fork differently when it is applied to one side of the skull or sternum compared with the other, even though it is a single bone).

A small number of studies examined the value of these signs and found them to be too common in patients with disease to have much specificity. For example, in one study, 69 of 80 patients with organic disease were found to have midline splitting of vibration sense [32]. Midline splitting also occurs

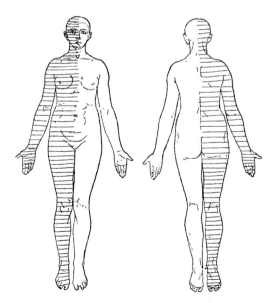

Fig. 4. A case of hemisensory disturbance depicted by Pierre Janet. (*From* Janet P, Raymond F. Nevroses et idées fixes. Paris: Felix Alcan; 1898.)

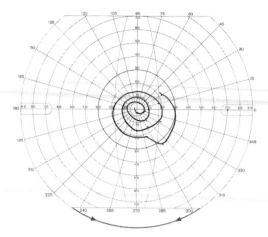

Fig. 5. Patients with functional visual symptoms often have spiral visual fields as shown here on this Goldmann visual perimetry chart. The spiral occurs as they see less and less peripherally as the test proceeds.

after thalamic stroke. There are other sensory signs, used mainly for patients complaining of anesthesia, but their validity has never been tested. These are not recommended in routine clinical practice but may have a role in medico-legal work or in patients of lower intelligence. Such tests include the following:

- Asking the patient to say "Yes" when they feel you touch them and "No" when they don't
- Testing hand sensation with the patient's fingers interlocked behind their back
- Asking the patient to close their eyes and touch their nose with the finger you touch

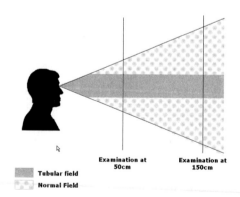

Fig. 6. A "tubular" field deficit is inconsistent with the laws of optics and eye physiology and is often found ipsilateral to functional hemisensory disturbance. Simply test visual fields at near and far distances (reproduced with permission of BMJ publications) [1].

A groundbreaking functional imaging study by Vuilleimier et al [33] has advanced knowledge about patients with hemisensory (and motor) symptoms. In one of the key parts of this study, four patients were imaged with SPECT while they were symptomatic and again when they had recovered. The scans showed hypofunction of the contralateral thalamus and basal ganglia during the symptomatic state relative to recovery (Fig. 7). Although this does not tell us why the problem was there or whether this appearance could be achieved simply by paying attention to a mild physiological asymmetry, it is in keeping with the idea of a functional hemisensory state. Studies such as this challenge us to broaden a purely psychogenic interpretation of functional symptoms to include biological and physiological factors. They also help us to explain the mechanism of the patient's symptoms to the patient as well as the multiple factors that may explain why that mechanism has occurred.

She Says She Is Not Depressed—But Is She?

In this case example, the patient has not only hemisensory symptoms but other symptoms common in this patient group, including fatigue, sleep disturbance (either too much or not enough), and concentration difficulties. These are, of course, somatic symptoms of depression. The patient also complains of marked loss of pleasure in doing things, all of which would qualify her for a DSM-IV diagnosis of current major depression. Typically, however, she is adamant that she is not depressed. If she had been asked if her symptoms got her down rather than was she feeling down, a different answer might have emerged. Framing the question in this way can remove an implication of blaming the patient for their problem.

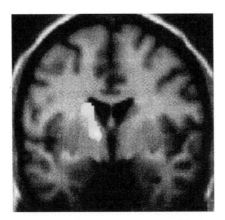

Fig. 7. Functional imaging study comparing appearances during the symptomatic state of four patients with unilateral functional sensory and motor disturbance with a subsequent scans after recovery. There was contralateral hypofunction of the basal ganglia and thalamus. (*From* Vuilleumier P, Chicherio C, Assal F, Schwartz S, Skusman D, Landis T. Functional neuroanatomical correlates of hysterical sensorimotor loss. Brain 2001;124:1077–90; with permission.)

What Is the Relevance of Her Feelings of Detachment?

The patient describes symptoms of depersonalization and derealization (symptoms that are placed under the broader banner of dissociation). This is the feeling of being detached or removed from your own body or your environment. Patients may simply describe this as feeling dizzy or weird and may be unable or unwilling to articulate the sensation further because they do not know how to describe it or because they fear they may be symptoms of "going crazy." Dissociative symptoms are common in neurologic disorders, especially epilepsy and migraine, and psychiatric disorders, such as panic disorder and depression. They also occur commonly in the general population, particularly in younger age groups. They do not have a great deal of diagnostic value but can be helpful to identify in a case like the one presented. Not only are patients often relieved to hear that the symptom does not mean they are going mad, but if there is a functional symptom, the presence of dissociation can be used to explain why they have the symptom ("It is the same detached feeling you experience all over your body, but just concentrated on one half"). Depersonalization and derealization do not respond well to medication. A cognitive behavioral approach to treatment for people who only have the symptom of depersonalization has been described [34].

So How Can All These Symptoms Be Put Together in a Way That Will Help Treatment?

The patient in case four has functional sensory symptoms, fatigue, sleep problems, anhedonia, and symptoms of depersonalization. Patients often have a mix of symptoms such as these. A neurologist does not need psychiatric training, or even take a psychiatric history from the patient, to be able to formulate these into a coherent form for the patient. For example, an explanation of the problem could start with a description of the vicious circle whereby pain interferes with sleep, which in turn leads to tiredness, which in turn leads to worse pain. Depersonalization can be said to be a consequence of fatigue and low mood a consequence of the whole symptom complex. Functional sensory symptoms can be explained as arising from an altered brain state that the patient is in as the result of their illness. This is often an overly simplistic approach, but it can be a good start for a patient in bewilderment with multiple symptoms. It also potentially makes more sense of subsequent interventions (eg, improving sleep and pain with medication, asking for psychological help with low mood).

Case 5: Prolonged Unconsciousness

A 27-year-old woman is admitted to gynecology for a termination of pregnancy. The procedure is straightforward, but afterward the anesthetist is surprised to find that the patient does not regain consciousness. She has the appearances and vital signs of someone who is asleep but cannot be woken up. Several hours pass with no change. A neurologist is called to make an assessment.

How Would You Assess This Patient and Confirm a Suspicion of Functional Coma?

In this case, the admitting gynecology team was not aware of the patient's extensive psychiatric history, with episodes of self-harm, depression, and a probable personality disorder on a background of childhood abuse. There had also been a similar episode 2 years ago that had lasted 8 days.

Physical examination in a case like this involves a standard coma assessment, looking carefully for signs useful in functional coma. These include

- Resistance against eye opening
- Response to painful stimuli (patients may be surprisingly unresponsive to nail bed or sternal pressure). Touching the inside of the nostril with a vibrating 1024Hz tuning fork is a particularly intense and surprising (but harmless) stimulus [35].
- Allowing the hand to drop from a height and observing the rate of descent. Transient retention of tone in this situation is much more useful than seeing if it drops on the patient's face, which should not be encouraged.
- Careful observation for states of normal sleep superimposed on the coma

An event such as this is rare and will normally resolve spontaneously in time. In some situations, if the patient is at risk from immobility, the authors have used sedation to, paradoxically, wake up the patient and trigger a recovery.

Summary

In this series of case vignettes, the authors have emphasized that the diagnosis of functional symptoms should normally rest on the presence of positive evidence of the problem being functional rather than the absence of evidence of organic disease. In addition, practitioners should be prepared to make a functional diagnosis in a patient who also has evidence of disease. Misdiagnosis of functional symptoms occurs no more than for other neurological and psychiatric disorders. The neurologist has an important role in being able to transmit the diagnosis in a way that will not offend the patient but will also facilitate recovery. The key elements of this explanation are making the patient feel believed and emphasizing potential reversibility. A multidisciplinary approach involving concurrent physical and psychological treatments is often recommended, although further study is required to determine the best approaches to explain and treat these conditions.

References

[1] Stone J, Carson A, Sharpe M. Functional symptoms and signs in neurology: assessment and diagnosis. J Neurol Neurosurg Psychiatry 2005;76(Suppl 1):i2–12.

[2] Stone J, Carson A, Sharpe M. Functional symptoms in neurology: management. J Neurol Neurosurg Psychiatry 2005;76(Suppl 1):i13–21.

[3] Reuber M, Elger CE. Psychogenic nonepileptic seizures: a review and update. Epilepsy Behav 2003;4:205–16.

[4] Cuthill FM, Espie CA. Sensitivity and specificity of procedures for the differential diagnosis of epileptic and non-epileptic seizures: a systematic review. Seizure 2005;14(5):293–303.

[5] McGonigal A, Oto M, Russell AJ, Greene J, Duncan R. Outpatient video EEG recording in the diagnosis of non-epileptic seizures: a randomised controlled trial of simple suggestion techniques. J Neurol Neurosurg Psychiatry 2002;72(4):549–51.

[6] Chen DK, So YT, Fisher RS. Use of serum prolactin in diagnosing epileptic seizures: report of the Therapeutics and Technology Assessment Subcommittee of the American Academy of Neurology. Neurology 2005;65(5):668–75.

[7] Oribe E, Amini R, Nissenbaum E, Boal B. Serum prolactin concentrations are elevated after syncope. Neurology 1996;47(1):60–2.

[8] Alving J. Serum prolactin levels are elevated also after pseudo-epileptic seizures. Seizure 1998;7(2):85–9.

[9] Stone J, Binzer M, Sharpe M. Illness beliefs and locus of control: a comparison of patients with pseudoseizures and epilepsy. J Psychosom Res 2004;57(6):541–7.

[10] Stone J, Campbell K, Sharma N, Carson A, Warlow CP, Sharpe M. What should we call pseudoseizures? The patient's perspective. Seizure 2003;12(8):568–72.

[11] Carton S, Thompson PJ, Duncan JS. Non-epileptic seizures: patients' understanding and reaction to the diagnosis and impact on outcome. Seizure 2003;12(5):287–94.

[12] Oto M, Espie C, Pelosi A, Selkirk M, Duncan R. Safety of antiepileptic drug withdrawal in patients with non-epileptic seizures. J Neurol Neurosurg Psychiatry 2005;76(12):1682–5.

[13] O'Malley PG, Jackson JL, Santoro J, Tomkins G, Balden E, Kroenke K. Antidepressant therapy for unexplained symptoms and symptom syndromes. J Fam Pract 1999;48(12): 980–90.

[14] Kroenke K, Swindle R. Cognitive-behavioral therapy for somatization and symptom syndromes: a critical review of controlled clinical trials. Psychother Psychosom 2000;69(4): 205–15.

[15] Goldstein LH, Deale AC, Mitchell-O'Malley SJ, Toone BK, Mellers JD. An evaluation of cognitive behavioral therapy as a treatment for dissociative seizures: a pilot study. Cogn Behav Neurol 2004;17(1):41–9.

[16] Stone J, Zeman A, Sharpe M. Functional weakness and sensory disturbance. J Neurol Neurosurg Psychiatry 2002;73(3):241–5.

[17] Sonoo M. Abductor sign: a reliable new sign to detect unilateral non-organic paresis of the lower limb. J Neurol Neurosurg Psychiatry 2004;73:121–5.

[18] Todd RB. Clinical lectures on paralyses. diseases of the brain, and other affections of the nervous system. London: Churchill; 1854.

[19] Charcot J-M. Nouvelle Iconographie de Salpêtrière. Clinique des maladies du systeme verveux. Publiée sous la direction du par Paul Richer, Gilles de la Tourette, Albert Londe; 1888.

[20] Gould R, Miller BL, Goldberg MA, Benson DF. The validity of hysterical signs and symptoms. J Nerv Ment Dis 1986;174(10):593–7.

[21] Slater ET, Glithero E. A follow-up of patients diagnosed as suffering from "hysteria." J Psychosom Res 1965;9(1):9–13.

[22] Stone J, Smyth R, Carson A, Lewis SC, Prescott R, Warlow C, et al. The misdiagnosis of conversion symptoms/hysteria: a systematic review. BMJ 2005;331(7523):989.

[23] Schrag A, Trimble M, Quinn N, Bhatia K. The syndrome of fixed dystonia: an evaluation of 103 patients. Brain 2004;127(Pt 10):2360–72.

[24] Fahn S, Williams DT. Psychogenic dystonia. Adv Neurol 1988;50:431–55.

[25] Thomas M, Jankovic J. Psychogenic movement disorders: diagnosis and management. CNS Drugs 2004;18(7):437–52.

[26] Schrag A, Lang AE. Psychogenic movement disorders. Curr Opin Neurol 2005;18(4): 399–404.

[27] Hallett M, Cloninger CR, Fahn S, Jankovic J, Lang AE, Yudofsky S. Psychogenic movement disorders. Philadelphia: Lippincott, Williams and Wilkins and the American Academy of Neurology; 2005.

[28] Edwards MJ, Trikouli E, Martino D, Bozi M, Dale RC, Church AJ, et al. Anti-basal ganglia antibodies in patients with atypical dystonia and tics: a prospective study. Neurology 2004; 63(1):156–8.

[29] Verdugo RJ, Ochoa JL. Abnormal movements in complex regional pain syndrome: assessment of their nature. Muscle Nerve 2000;23(2):198–205.

[30] Toth C. Hemisensory syndrome is associated with a low diagnostic yield and a nearly uniform benign prognosis. J Neurol Neurosurg Psychiatry 2003;74(8):1113–6.

[31] Beatty S. Non-organic visual loss. Postgrad Med J 1999;75(882):201–7.

[32] Rolak LA. Psychogenic sensory loss. J Nerv Ment Dis 1988;176(11):686–7.

[33] Vuilleumier P, Chicherio C, Assal F, Schwartz S, Skusman D, Landis T. Functional neuroanatomical correlates of hysterical sensorimotor loss. Brain 2001;124:1077–90.

[34] Hunter EC, Baker D, Phillips ML, Sierra M, David AS. Cognitive-behaviour therapy for depersonalisation disorder: an open study. Behav Res Ther 2005;43(9):1121–30.

[35] Harvey P. Harvey's 1 and 2. Pract Neurol 2004;4(3):178–9.

ELSEVIER
SAUNDERS

Neurol Clin 24 (2006) 405–412

NEUROLOGIC
CLINICS

Index

Note: Page numbers of article titles are in **boldface** type.

0733-8619/06/$ - see front matter © 2006 Elsevier Inc. All rights reserved.
doi:10.1016/S0733-8619(06)00045-4

Changing Your Address?

Make sure your subscription changes too! When you notify us of your new address, you can help make our job easier by including an exact copy of your Clinics label number with your old address (see illustration below.) This number identifies you to our computer system and will speed the processing of your address change. Please be sure this label number accompanies your old address and your corrected address—you can send an old Clinics label with your number on it or just copy it exactly and send it to the address listed below.

We appreciate your help in our attempt to give you continuous coverage. Thank you.

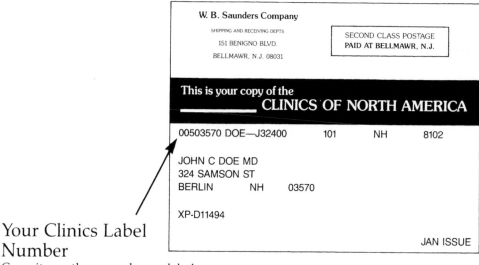

Your Clinics Label Number

Copy it exactly or send your label along with your address to:
Elsevier Periodicals Customer Service
6277 Sea Harbor Drive
Orlando, FL 32887-4800
Call Toll Free 1-800-654-2452

Please allow four to six weeks for delivery of new subscriptions and for processing address changes.